THE ARTHROPATHIES

A Handbook of Roentgen Diagnosis

THE HANDBOOKS OF
ROENTGEN DIAGNOSIS

THE ARTHROPATHIES: A. A. de LORIMIER, M.D., *Colonel (MC)*
U. S. Army; Commandant, The Army School of Roentgenology, Memphis, Tenn.

THE CHEST: LEO G. RIGLER, M.D., *Professor of Radiology,*
University of Minnesota Medical School and Graduate School of Medicine.

THE GASTRO-INTESTINAL TRACT: FRED JENNER HODGES, M.D.,
Professor of Roentgenology, University of Michigan Medical School.

THE OSSEOUS SYSTEM: VINCENT W. ARCHER, M.D.,
Professor of Roentgenology, University of Virginia Department of Medicine.

THE SKULL, SINUSES & MASTOIDS: KARL KORNBLUM, M.D.,
Clinical Professor of Radiology, University of Pennsylvania School of Medicine.

THE URINARY TRACT: H. DABNEY KERR, M.D., *Professor of*
Radiology, and CARL L. GILLIES, M.D., *Associate Professor of Radiology,*
State University of Iowa College of Medicine.

THE
ARTHROPATHIES

A Handbook of
ROENTGEN DIAGNOSIS

by

ALFRED A. de LORIMIER, A.B.; M.A.; M.D.

Colonel, Medical Corps, United States Army; Commandant, The Army School of Roentgenology, Memphis, Tenn. Formerly Director, Department of Roentgenology, Army Medical School, Washington, D. C.

THE YEAR BOOK PUBLISHERS · INC.

304 South Dearborn Street · Chicago

DEDICATED TO ALL DOCTORS
POSSESSED OF SCIENTIFIC ENTHUSIASM
HAVING PRIMARY INTEREST IN THE PATIENT
SECONDARY BUT CLOSELY EQUIVALENT
INTEREST IN THE UNDERLYING PATHOLOGY
AND LEAST INTEREST IN THEIR PERSONAL GAIN
IN HANDLING THE CASE
DOCTORS EXERCISING THE STALWART
PROFESSIONAL PRINCIPLES OF
DR. L. L. STANLEY OF SAN RAFAEL, CALIFORNIA

Foreword

THIS BOOK reflects and fulfils the earnest wish of a man to serve his profession and his fellow-men. With the freely acknowledged aid of his able staff and many friends in civilian practice, Col. de Lorimier has drafted the worthwhile facts about the radiologic diagnosis of joint disease from the common store of knowledge and his own experience as a teacher of radiology and has marshaled them in orderly ranks, not for dress parade but for action in the field. This aim is clear, for nowhere in the book is there any padding or self-conscious rhetoric that would suggest a greater interest in ornamental diction than in useful data. Especially striking is the uniform presentation of the individual features of every arthropathy, in the same sequence with conspicuous headings, so that particular aspects of different diseases can readily be compared. Indeed, to many of us who had to learn about joint disease the hard way, by trial and error, this volume seems like a faithful robot that should guide even a novice. Let it not be supposed, however, that the author entertains any thought of making competent radiologists out of novices in a short time at the Army School with this book or by any other means. On the contrary, while he realizes the present necessity of intensive training, he insists that the training be as prolonged and as thorough as circumstances will permit.

Of the author himself, there is scarcely need to speak further. A valued contributor to radiologic literature, respected by his colleagues in the Army and by civilian radiologists, designer of the radiologic field equipment now in use by the Army, head of the Army School of Roentgenology, Col. de Lorimier holds a high place in the radiologic world. With such a background, the text that he has sponsored should have unusual merits and should serve its purpose with distinction.

B. R. KIRKLIN, M.D., *Colonel,* (*M.C.*)
Senior X-Ray Consultant, S.G.O., U. S. A.

Foreword

In the introduction to the discussion of abnormalities and diseases of the joints Colonel de Lorimier has outlined simply yet clearly the basic principles which should govern roentgenologic study and diagnosis as a whole. The importance of the author's insistence that conclusions drawn in each case should be based on an analytical study of the tangible evidence exhibited in the particular film under examination cannot be overemphasized.

It is equally important that the roentgenologist should not be denied the assistance of the corroborative clinical and laboratory data which frequently will give him a lead that may enable him to institute search for and visualize strictly roentgenologic criteria which might otherwise be overlooked. It might be offered as a constructive criticism that, in the conduct of the Department of Roentgenology in the average large hospital, the roentgenologist does not insist that sufficient time and opportunity be afforded him for an adequate study of the clinical data pertaining to each case.

Colonel de Lorimier's long experience as a student and teacher of roentgenology has enabled him to evaluate the relative importance of the strictly roentgenologic criteria and corroborative clinical data and to blend these into a practical working formula.

In order to present to its best advantage this concept of the x-ray and clinical data requisite to a proper roentgenologic diagnosis, the author has evolved the arrangement of subject matter as depicted in the text. In reality this is not a new classification, as Colonel de Lorimier somewhat apologetically states, but is a most practical and valuable grouping of the various clinical entities which produce similar roentgenologic characteristics.

Under the general heading of Juvenile Osteochondropathy are included those closely related clinical entities such as Legg-Perthes' disease or coxa plana, Osgood-Schlatter's disease of the tibial tuberosity and Köhler's disease of the tarsal-scaphoid. The whole group, with essential similarities and differences, is simultaneously placed before the student on a single mental photographic plate.

Among the many other valuable contributions is the statement that it is the roentgenologist's responsibility to consider an essential etiologic basis for the roentgenologic changes. The presence of hyperostotic changes along the joint margins should not be dismissed with a simple diagnosis of hypertrophic arthritis, for the condition may be due to many causes. Accidental or occupational trauma, faulty mechanics in weight-bearing and infections, as well as the degenerative changes of old age, may be the etiologic agent. Evaluation of the relative importance of each is often important in determining the type of treatment or the medicolegal liability.

This concept of presenting the varied data essential to the problem of roentgenologic diagnosis appears not only fundamental from a scientific standpoint but practicable for purposes of teaching roentgenology to the medical student and clinician.

J. S. SPEED, M.D.
Professor of Orthopedic Surgery
University of Tennessee

Preface

THIS HANDBOOK is a compilation of lectures presented since 1938 to officers at the Army Medical School, Washington, and the Army School of Roentgenology, Memphis. These lectures grew out of research and clinical interests initiated in 1932 by Col. John J. Moore. The material is presented in the form followed in our teaching. Instruction has been graphic, presenting first an orientation of the subject; then a catalogue, by films or lantern slides, of essential diagnostic roentgen criteria, and finally corroborative clinical and laboratory aspects. These lectures have been compiled with the assistance of many who, because of limitations of space, cannot be identified with each contribution. Our officer-students have given interesting films and stimulating professional opinions.

Especial thanks are due Col. William L. Thompson for his paternal interest and his generous tolerance of our weekly student conferences and for making available material from the x-ray clinic of Walter Reed General Hospital. Likewise, we are deeply indebted to Col. Henry W. Grady and Lieut. Col. Henry G. Moehring; the latter has selected and sent our school scores of invaluable films. Dr. George H. Hess, Uniontown, Pa., loaned several spine studies of coal miners, depicting spondyl-osteo-arthropathies. Dr. Henry L. Jaffe, New York City, made available studies of well established cases of osteoid osteoma and benign chondromyxoma. Dr. Edward B. D. Neuhauser, Boston, loaned various examples of congenital syphilis, rickets and scurvy. Dr. A. L. L. Bell, Brooklyn, loaned films on caisson disease; Dr. Harrison L. Martland, Newark, N. J., examples of radiation necrosis, as did also Commander Harold W. Jacox and Dr. Lester M. J. Friedman, from studies at the University of Michigan. Dr. Howard P. Doub, Detroit, loaned films on intervertebral tuberculosis; Dr. J. Robert Andrews, several studies of chordoma; Dr. J. N. Kimball, Takoma Park, Md., a case of synovioma and examples of developmental malformations. Lieut. E. G.

Dyer contributed films of juvenile rheumatoid arthritis. Lieut. Col. Paul V. McCarthy, Lieut. Col. Harold O. Brown and Maj. R. C. Massengill have sent scores of valuable studies. Dr. Charles Gottlieb, New York City, sent examples of chronic proliferative periostitis; Col. Bradley L. Coley, New York, one of the studies of hemorrhage in the joint; Maj. George R. Krause, one of persistent notochord; Maj. E. W. Egbert, the one of recurrent dislocation of the shoulder with the grooved defect; Maj. Raphael Pomeranz, the synovioma with erosion of the sacrum. Maj. Ernest P. Griffin and Capt. Everett L. Pirkey contributed a number of studies. Dr. Marcy L. Sussman, New York City, loaned the films on scleroderma; Dr. Fred Y. Kuhlman, Port Arthur, Tex., that of vertebra plana; Dr. Fred Coe, Washington, D. C., that of pseudarthrosis of the clavicles; Dr. Russell H. Morgan, Chicago, that of nephritic edema. Capt. Harold N. Neu obtained various examples of spinal malformations; Capt. John L. Gompertz, an example of localized osteomyelitis regional to the joint; Lieut. T. B. Bolitho, the interesting study of joint changes in sickle cell anemia; Capt. Hugh H. Hopkins, that of juvenile osteochondropathy of the scapular heads. Maj. A. C. Galluccio sent the studies of dissecans osteochondropathy involving the talus; Lieut. Col. Joseph Linsman, that of the spine in chronic fluoride poisoning. Maj. U. R. Ulferts sent several of the cases of healed rheumatoid arthritis, and Capt. P. A. Robins, one of the cases of osteochondropathy of the tarsal navicular. Dr. J. S. Speed, Dr. H. B. Boyd and the staff of the Willis C. Campbell Orthopedic Clinic, Memphis, have loaned scores of instructive cases; particular thanks are due for three of the cases of syphilitic arthritis and two of the osteochondropathies of the hip.

All have demonstrated scientific philanthropy by their cooperation with our teaching program and by their willingness that reproductions of their films be included here. If there are oversights in expressing this personal appreciation, apologies are sincerely offered.

Appreciation is expressed to Mr. H. A. Simons and the staff of the Year Book Publishers for their careful work in converting this lecture material into book form.

The importance of this phase of roentgenology cannot be overestimated when it is realized that the arthropathies have accounted for the third largest group of conditions requiring hospitalization and compensation since World War I. Since the present mobilization, they are constituting the fifth largest group requiring such care and pension.

—A. A. DE L.

Table of Contents

Introduction

As with any phase of roentgenology, an evaluation of the roentgen
evidence concerned with conditions in and about joints is dependent
on: (1) a substantial knowledge of embryology and the deviations
from normal development which might occur during prenatal life;
(2) an understanding of detailed anatomic relations, including topo-
graphic aspects; (3) a knowledge of pathologic changes together
with the roentgenographic features—the criteria which depict one or
another disease entity, and finally (4) familiarity with the clinical
aspects of the particular case, including laboratory findings. In addition to these more strictly doctor-requirements, the roentgenologist
must possess a knowledge of physical fundamentals which might
serve to guide him in adequately visualizing all of the various tissue
densities.

A high quality roentgenogram may be described as one containing
the maximum of detail with the optimum of contrast, the optimum
of radiographic density and the minimum of distortion. Not infre-
quently, the technical factors which are used result in such an
extreme degree of contrast that practically no visualization of the
soft tissues remains, or, if the soft tissues are visualized, the bones
appear as solid pieces of ivory, there being no architectural detail.
Too often does one accept mere visualization of the skeleton! This
probably accounts for the rather prevalent expression that there are
only two types of arthritis: "atrophic" and "hypertrophic." Too
many doctors appear to have been satisfied to limit their considerations to the condition of the bones. It is very certain that thereby
early stages of joint lesions are unrecognized.

In order to provide for recognition of abnormality in any stage, it
is definitely necessary to utilize roentgenographic technical factors
which accomplish visualization of the soft tissues as well as of the
osseous architecture—and an adequacy of visualization of all tissues

regardless of inflammation, exudation or other conditions leading to fogging of detail.

It is not possible to include in this text a detailed discussion of the technical factors concerned with detail, contrast, radiographic density and distortion. These are basic fundamentals described in any text on roentgenography. It is important, though, to emphasize the value of using cardboard holders (i.e., film envelopes), rather than cassettes with intensifying screens, whenever possible. (This does not dispute the fact that use of cassettes may be indicated even for thin parts when visualization of bone densities alone is desired.) Such a practice provides for greater sharpness of detail and a longer scale in the gradation of densities (i.e., reduction in contrast) and therefore more complete visualization of soft tissues, fascial planes and, at the same time, visualization of the osseous architecture. For the past 10 years, it has been the practice at the Army Medical School and the Army School of Roentgenology to use cardboard holders or light protective envelopes, rather than cassettes with intensifying screens, for all parts having thickness less than 10 cm. For certain cases, when special considerations warrant, this type of film holder is used even for parts having thickness greater than 10 cm. and even though a grid (i.e., stationary or Potter-Bucky diaphragm type) be required to counteract the effects of secondary radiation.

It is important, too, to emphasize the attributes of relatively long focal film distance. Unless the factor, distortion, is to be utilized for magnifying one or another portion of a joint, it is recommended that for the smaller joints of the extremities, the focal film distance be no less than 30 in.; for the joints of the trunk, that it be no less than 36 to 40 in. Relatively long focal film distance is another factor contributing to sharpness of detail.

It is rather common practice to use the lowest possible kilovoltage. Such a policy is detrimental. High kilovoltage provides for a relatively long scale in the gradation of densities. It serves to counteract contrast. Today, the film manufacturers have developed for us emulsions and processing chemicals which produce a high degree of contrast; the equipment manufacturers have developed x-ray machines which tolerate high milliamperage loads, tempting one to reduce the kilovoltage and thereby increase the contrast; and the

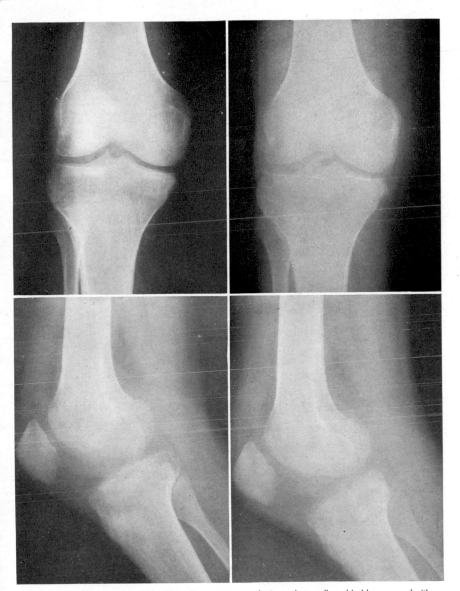

Fig. 1 (left above).—Low kilovoltage. The part measured 12 cm., but cardboard holder was used with grid (5:1 ratio, moving type). Factors: 66 kv.p., 210 ma.s., at 30 in. Failure to visualize soft tissues due to excessive contrast. Greater contrast would have been obtained had intensifying screens been used. **Fig. 2 (right above).**—Same case. High kilovoltage. Same conditions except 91 kv.p., 20 ma.s. Greater gradation of densities—note visualization of soft tissues *and* osseous architecture. Higher kilovoltage is especially advantageous with intensifying screens. **Fig. 3 (left below).**—Same case. Low kilovoltage. Same conditions except 63 kv.p., 210 ma.s. **Fig. 4 (right below).**—Same case. High kilovoltage. Same conditions except 90 kv.p., 20 ma.s. Improved visualization of soft tissues and osseous architecture.

intensifying screen manufacturers have developed "fast" screens which likewise tempt one to reduce the kilovoltage. With all these influences, there is a definite tendency to obtain too great a degree of contrast. The manufacturers' developments are helpful, but they should be utilized properly. They require use of kilovoltages greater than those used by many, in order to avoid multiplying contrast to the degree of *reductio ad absurdum.*

High kilovoltage is favorable not only because it widens the scale of radiographic densities but also because inherently it provides for reduction of exposure time. When cassettes with intensifying screens must be used this is particularly true, for the higher the kilovoltage the greater the intensity of their fluorescence.

The sensitization curve with regard to the kilovoltage factor and intensifying screen fluorescence must be respected. The higher the kilovoltage, the "faster" the intensifying screen effect. No one "speed factor" should be assigned to a cassette. The speed varies markedly in proportion to the kilovoltage. Therefore, it is recommended that a calibration curve be sketched on the back of each cassette so as to provide for the proper compensation by reduction of milliampere-seconds, with increment steps of kilovoltage. Otherwise, the roentgenograms will be of uncertain radiographic densities and too many of them will have excessive densities. Excessive radiographic density, of course, obscures detail, particularly soft tissue detail.

For the joints of the extremities, particularly when using cassettes, it has been found practical to vary the kilovoltage from 50 to 90, depending on the thickness of the part. Paradoxical as it may seem, though, for thicker parts such as the spine, it is better to limit the kilovoltage to the 70–85 kv.p. range. This is particularly true with respect to the lower thoracic and the lumbosacral spine, where the density and dimensions of the tissues are responsible for the production of a great intensity of secondary radiation.

Secondary radiation prevents suitable sharpness of detail. Its intensity in the direction of the film is increased proportionately in accordance with the kilovoltage, the prolongation of milliampere-seconds and the volume and density of tissue exposed. As already mentioned, the grid should be used for filtering these rays whenever their intensities would result in perceptible fogging. A cone or a

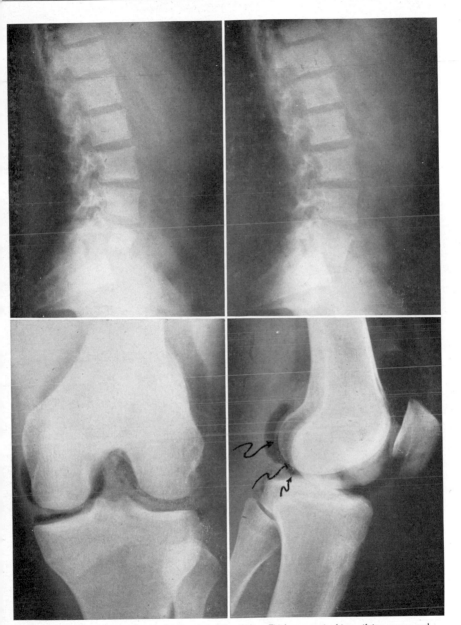

Fig. 5 (left above).—Lumbosacral spine. Low kilovoltage. Thickness required intensifying screens and grid. Factors: 72 kv.p., 700 ma.s., at 40 in. **Fig. 6 (right above).**—Same case. High kilovoltage: 90 kv.p., 140 ma.s. Note fogginess due to increased secondary radiation. **Fig. 7 (left below).**—Pneumo-arthrography, P-A projection, with leg slightly flexed. Menisci and cruciate ligament outlined. Stereoscopy with this technic is especially informative. **Fig. 8 (right below).**—Pneumo-arthrography. Articular cartilages, usually ray transparent, visualized by contrast provided by air.

diaphragm may be placed over the part to limit the area of coverage by the primary beam. It may be practical to use either of these even with the grid when the latter does not sufficiently eliminate the secondary fog.

With proper roentgenographic technic, it is possible to consider practically all the tissues in or about joints. A routine analysis should include the following aspects:

1. The soft tissues: What is the condition of the musculature? Is there evidence of atrophy? Are tendons or muscle bundles deviated from their normal positions? Do the vessels indicate age by calcific streaking of the arteries? Are phleboliths visualized? Are the fascial planes distinct or are they obliterated because of inflammation or edema? Are there any abnormal tumefactions?

2. The regional bones (i.e., at a distance from the joint): Are there any abnormalities of contour? Is the periosteum visualized? Is the periosteum separated, as by hemorrhage, or is there evidence of its proliferation? What is the condition of the osseous architecture? Is there evidence of delayed ossification; of deossification? Is there an actual erosion or sequestration? Is there evidence of superimposed calcification or hyperostosis?

3. The articular cortexes (i.e., the extremities of the bones regional to the joints): Is there evidence of sclerosis (eburnation)? Is there any depletion of these portions? Are there marginal or intra-articular spur formations? What is the condition of the osseous articular surfaces—are they smooth or irregular, of normal convexity or concavity, or are they flattened?

4. The articular cartilages (being ray transparent under ordinary conditions, an evaluation must be made by indirect evidence): Is fibrillation or compression of cartilage indicated by spur formations around the osseous articular cortexes? Is it indicated by narrowing of the joint space? Are there indications of loss of cushioning of the bones by eburnations of the articular cortexes? Is there evidence of actual calcification in the cartilage? Is there any indication of destruction of it, i.e., by fibrous or osseous ankyloses? Should air or oxygen be injected into the joint (see Figs. 7 and 8) to provide intra-articular contrast and actual visualization of the cartilage (pneumo-arthrography)?

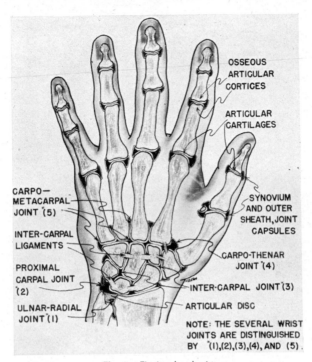

OSSEOUS
ARTICULAR
CORTICES

ARTICULAR
CARTILAGES

CARPO—
METACARPAL
JOINT (5)

INTER-CARPAL
LIGAMENTS

PROXIMAL
CARPAL JOINT
(2)

ULNAR-RADIAL
JOINT (1)

SYNOVIUM
AND OUTER
SHEATH, JOINT
CAPSULES

CARPO-THENAR
JOINT (4)

INTER-CARPAL JOINT (3)

ARTICULAR DISC

NOTE: THE SEVERAL WRIST
JOINTS ARE DISTINGUISHED
BY (1),(2),(3),(4), AND (5).

Fig. 9.—The hand and wrist.

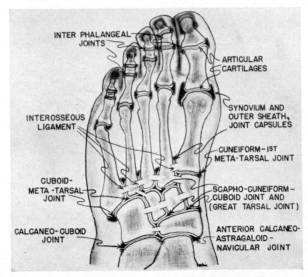

INTER PHALANGEAL
JOINTS

INTEROSSEOUS
LIGAMENT

CUBOID-
META-TARSAL
JOINT

CALGANEO-CUBOID
JOINT

ARTICULAR
CARTILAGES

SYNOVIUM AND
OUTER SHEATH,
JOINT CAPSULES

CUNEIFORM—IST
META-TARSAL JOINT

SCAPHO-CUNEIFORM—
CUBOID JOINT AND
(GREAT TARSAL JOINT)

ANTERIOR CALCANEO-
ASTRAGALOID-
NAVICULAR JOINT

Fig. 10.—The foot. Plantar semilateral projection.

5. The synovial membrane and joint capsule (being ray transparent under ordinary conditions, an evaluation must be made indirectly): Is there evidence of effusion (transudate, exudate or hemorrhage), as indicated by widening of the joint space? Is villous or pannus coverage suggested because of close apposition of the articular cortexes and the formation of a "cleavage line" (indicating fibrous ankylosis)? Are "millet seed" ossifications present, indicating villous hypertrophy? Is there any evidence of actual lineal calcification?

6. The joint space (including not only the spacing between the osseous articular cortexes but also the larger volume located beyond the borders of the articular surfaces): Is there widening? Is there deviation of regional soft tissues? Are there any ray-opaque inclusions ("joint mice")?

All these considerations must be based on tangible evidence. This evidence may be direct or indirect. However, the entire study must be scientifically accomplished. It must be analytical. One must not base a diagnosis on a recollection of a "picture" of this or of that condition. Unless tangible features—criteria—can be discerned, comments are too likely to be unreliable and superficial. A surgical confrere once defined a roentgenologist as "a bird with a distorted imagination." Too many doctors believe this because they think that roentgenologists depend on recognizing pictures of pathologic conditions—as they would recognize a photograph of a relative or friend. Even though one has had long practice in this specialty, it is important routinely to enforce at least a mental listing of the *criteria* which are actually visualized in each case and then to consider the possible conditions in which such criteria might be found. As a consultant, the roentgenologist is entitled to know the clinical aspects as well as corroborative laboratory findings. However, he should not start with these, for he might then be too greatly tempted to read into the film preconceived ideas.

Following this policy, the presentations which follow have been arranged so that *roentgen criteria*—not imaginative, but actually visible criteria—are listed first. Thereafter, there are presented suggestions regarding corroborative x-ray evidence which might possibly be found in other portions of the body. Then, there is a discus-

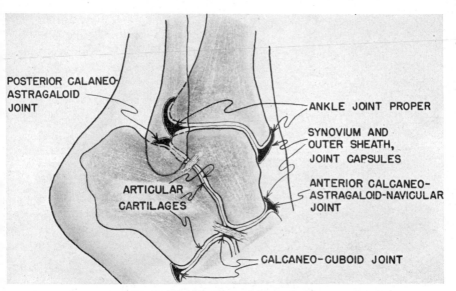

Fig. 11.—The ankle. Plantar oblique projection.

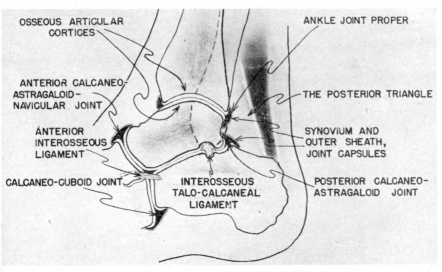

Fig. 12.—The ankle. Lateral projection.

sion of the likelihood of the condition occurring at one or another age, in one or the other sex, perhaps in one or another race or particular occupation, etc. Finally, high points pertaining to a typical history or a typical physical examination are suggested. These aspects are limited to what might serve for direct or specific questioning by the roentgenologist. Likewise, consideration has been given to supportive laboratory tests—tests which might already have been accomplished or which might be suggested by the roentgenologist.

Such should be the trend of thinking by the doctor who is faced with one, two or a few films made by exposures of one or a few parts of a patient of whom, likely, he has never seen or heard before. A trustworthy roentgenologic diagnosis must depend on a correlation of the clinical aspects and other special studies with the roentgenographic evidence.

It is essential that these problems be attacked with an open and scientific mind and that a range of diagnostic possibilities be considered. In many cases it is dangerous to concentrate one's thinking on a single entity. Such a tendency can be obviated by making a mental list of the possibilities. This calls for a classification. Classifications of lesions of the joints are numerous, and it is risky to suggest a new one. Some are based on bacteriologic considerations; some, on pathologic changes; others, entirely on morphologic findings. All seem to have their shortcomings.

Usually, a condition cannot be improved unless its *cause* is recognized. Unfortunately, with lesions of the joints, as Nichols and Richardson have pointed out: "Each type represents reaction of the joint tissues to a considerable variety of causes." So-called "mixed types" are numerous. In particular, the effects of trauma are likely to be superimposed on other changes. This factor is, of course, basic to the changes which occur after violent injury. It is largely responsible for the osteo-arthropathy of old age, the hypertrophic changes following hemorrhage and the changes in Charcot joints. These changes may also be found after subsidence of acute episodes in "rheumatoid arthritis" and even when an actual infection has existed within the joint (i.e., following true infectious arthritis). Surely, then, the mere presence of hyperostatic changes should not

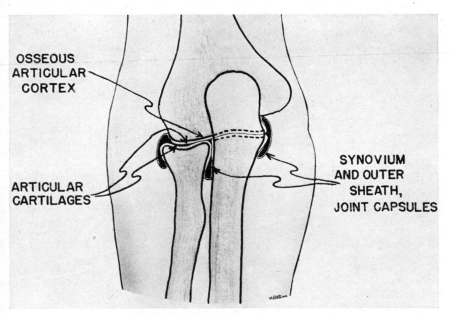

OSSEOUS
ARTICULAR
CORTEX

ARTICULAR
CARTILAGES

SYNOVIUM
AND OUTER
SHEATH,
JOINT CAPSULES

Fig. 13.—The elbow. Anteroposterior projection.

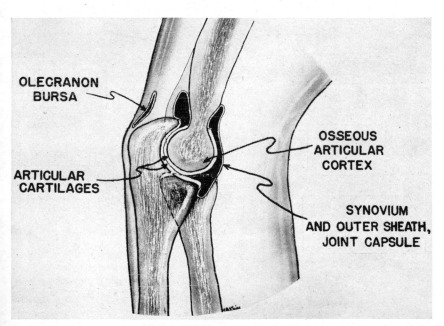

OLECRANON
BURSA

ARTICULAR
CARTILAGES

OSSEOUS
ARTICULAR
CORTEX

SYNOVIUM
AND OUTER SHEATH,
JOINT CAPSULE

Fig. 14.—The elbow. Lateral projection.

depict the condition as "hypertrophic arthritis," for all the afore-
mentioned types would be so called with, possibly, resultant loss of
time in proper handling of the patient. Therefore it is the roentgenologist's serious responsibility to search for the most indicative criteria and always to consider an essential *etiologic* basis for the
findings.

Guided by etiologic considerations the classification indicated in
the Table of Contents has been devised, and the subject matter of
this book is arranged in that order.

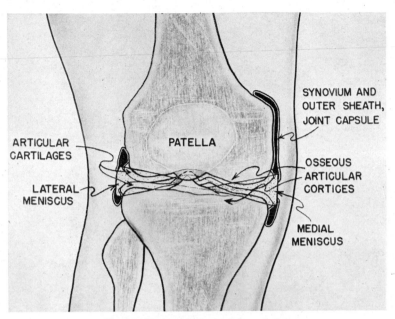

Fig. 15.—The knee. Postero-anterior projection.

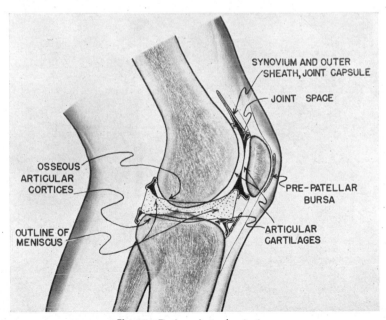

Fig. 16.—The knee. Lateral projection.

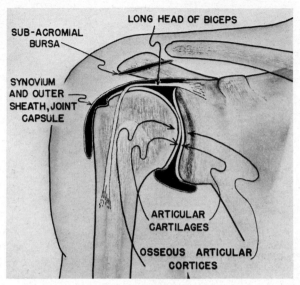

Fig. 17.—The shoulder.

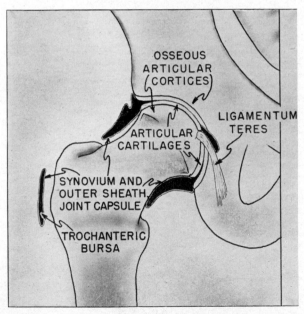

Fig. 18.—The hip.

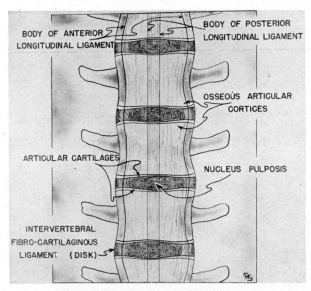

Fig. 19.—The spine. Anteroposterior projection.

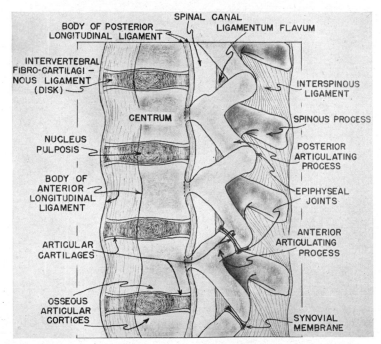

Fig. 20.—The spine. Lateral projection.

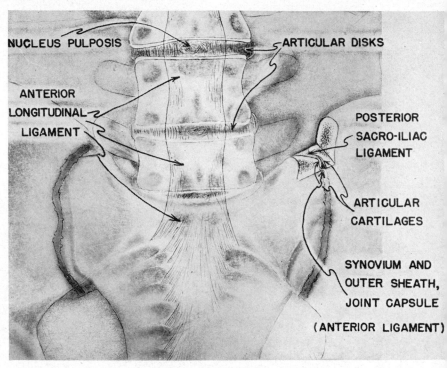

NUCLEUS PULPOSIS

ARTICULAR DISKS

ANTERIOR LONGITUDINAL LIGAMENT

POSTERIOR SACRO-ILIAC LIGAMENT

ARTICULAR CARTILAGES

SYNOVIUM AND OUTER SHEATH, JOINT CAPSULE (ANTERIOR LIGAMENT)

Fig. 21.—The sacro-iliac joints. Anteroposterior projection.

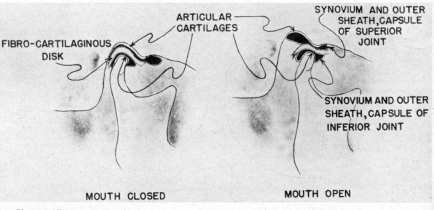

ARTICULAR CARTILAGES

SYNOVIUM AND OUTER SHEATH, CAPSULE OF SUPERIOR JOINT

FIBRO-CARTILAGINOUS DISK

SYNOVIUM AND OUTER SHEATH, CAPSULE OF INFERIOR JOINT

MOUTH CLOSED

MOUTH OPEN

Fig. 22.—The temporomandibular joint. Lateral projection; incident ray angled 33 degrees toward feet.

PART I

The Peripheral Joints

Normal Development, Malformations and Pathologic Changes in Peripheral Joints

AT TIMES, developmental malformations may be confused with disease states. Certainly for this reason the embryologic aspects of joint development are important. They are equally important for considering the detailed anatomic constituents of one and another of the joints, for with such knowledge a more adequate mental picture of truly pathologic derangements can be developed.

The structures of the peripheral joints are derived entirely from mesoderm. As early as the third week of intra-uterine life, the future bones and joints can be distinguished as cores of mesenchyme (scleroblastema) extending from the vertebral column more or less as axial rods in the limb buds. During the fifth and sixth weeks, because of condensations of cells in certain portions and the relative lack of cell multiplication between these portions, the cores develop the appearance of chains of mesenchymal links. A degree of segmentation is produced. Those portions consisting of the condensed cellular structures, the segments, are the progenitors of the bones, while the more loose intersegmental tissues develop into the joints.

If little or no movement is to occur between the bone-forming segments, the intersegmental tissues develop into ordinary fibrous tissue. They produce thereby merely a bridging of the bone ends or borders. This type of union is described as a *synarthrodial joint*. Normally, its complete form is not found in the extremities, though fibrous septations or interosseous ligaments do exist in the hip, knee, feet and wrists. The posterior half, or a greater portion, of the sacro-iliac joints is likewise of this type. However, the most typical example of a synarthrodial joint is the fixation of the bones of the cranium, where fibrous tissues alone intervene between their borders without articular cartilages, joint spacings or a joint capsule. The ribs are similarly

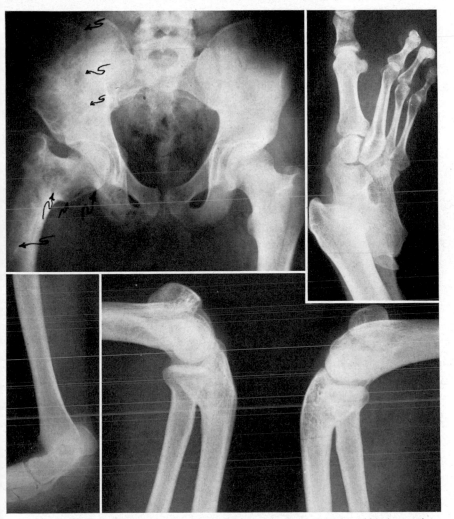

Abnormalities due to mesenchymal defects. **Fig. 23 (left above).**—Deformation of neck of the femur and cystic structure in ilium and femur, with femoral bowing and abnormal weight-bearing—attributed to abnormal metaplasia of the mesenchyme. This type is described as polyostotic fibrous dysplasia. **Fig. 24 (right above)** and **Fig. 25 (left below).**—Absence of cuneiforms, second metatarsal, phalanges and fibula, caused by lack of development of mesenchymal cords, progenitors of these bones. Result is deformity, abnormal weight-bearing and, eventually, static osteo-arthropathy. **Fig. 26 (right below).**—Fragmentations of olecranon processes of both ulnae, and bending with consequent abnormality of joint function—in a case of fragilitas osseum (osteogenesis imperfecta; osteopsathyrosis), attributable to abnormal mesenchymal development and transition.

fixed to the sternum, though with them, the intervening tissue is cartilage rather than fibrous tissue—the fixation therefore being described as a *synchondrosis*.

Where slightly greater joint function is required, the intersegmental mesenchymal tissues develop into fibrocartilage, thereby permitting at least a limited degree of movement. Such joints are described as *amphi-arthrodial* in type. This type of joint is normally not found in the extremities. The intervertebral disks of the spine are good examples.

For joints of definitely greater range of function, the intersegmental cells develop into more or less redundant loose tissue. Eventually this tissue produces a joint capsule. As such, two distinct layers are formed: an outer supporting layer, and an inner lining membrane. The outer layer provides support both because it is a complete jacket and because of the development in it of actual joint ligaments. The inner synovial layer provides lubrication for the articulating surfaces and, being highly vascular, also supplies a portion of the nourishment to the joint cartilages. Joints of this type, then, have a joint space. The extremities of the bones are contained within the capsular space. Normally, the actual articulating surfaces are composed of cartilage—the "articular cartilages." In the adult, the cartilages are simple caps fixed to the extremities of the bones. As with cartilage in general, they are ray transparent so that roentgenographically their thicknesses provide what is generally interpreted as joint space. Of course it must be realized that there is a contact apposition of the cartilaginous articular surfaces and that most of the joint spacing exists anteriorly and posteriorly to these contacts as well as to the sides of the extremities of the bones. Embryonically, the inner lining of the joint capsule, synovial membrane, extends over the surfaces of the articular cartilages, but with use of the joint it becomes obliterated over the actual areas of articulation, remaining fused with these cartilages at their peripheries. Such is the condition in *diarthrodial joints*, the most common type found in the extremities.

Where movement in more than one plane or where a rotary or gliding action is required, the diarthrodial type of joint is more elaborately developed. In addition to forming a joint capsule, the intersegmental tissues develop an intracapsular fibrocartilaginous

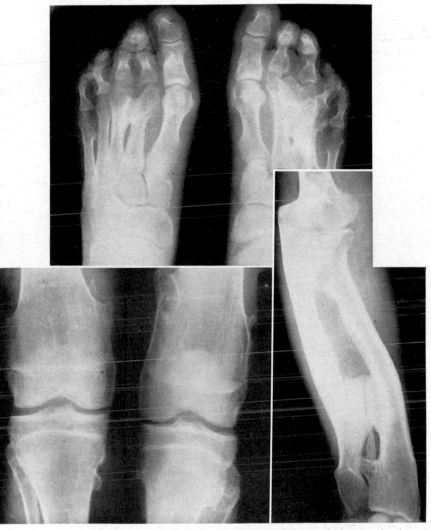

Limitation of joint function may be due to mechanical interference by osseous bridgings, as found in chondrodysplasia, as in **Figure 27 (above)** and **Figure 29 (right below)**; or, to a lesser extent, there may be limitation of motion because of interference with muscle and tendon function owing to exostoses **(Fig. 28, left below)**. Secondary changes of static osteo-arthropathy may develop. However, all of these findings are attributable to abnormal delimitation of the mesenchymal cords or transition into cartilage and then into bone.

plate. This is usually described as a disk or meniscus. It appears that it is intended to provide an auxiliary cushioning and support by filling marginal spacings around the regions of articulation. These disks are found in joints such as the knee, radio-ulnar and temporomandibular. They are *compound joints*.

Occasionally, there is abnormal development. For instance, the condensations of mesenchymal cells may develop more regularly than described, without segmentation, thereby defeating the requirements for separate bone formation. The result is absence of joint formation—described as a *synosteosis* or a *synarthrosis*. Thus, the three phalanges of a digit may be fused as one, the radius and ulna may be joined together or two ribs may be fused.

The entire skeleton is first composed of these mesenchymal condensations. In the case of the flat bones of the calvarium and some of those of the face, there is a direct transition of the mesenchymal tissues into bone. This is a relatively slow process, little of which is consummated during fetal life. Bones developed in this manner are described as "membranous bones." Except for the bones of the skull, the skeleton is developed by way of an intermediate stage of cartilage.

The metaplasia concerned with this intermediate stage occurs as early as the second fetal month. Transition, either directly from the mesenchyme or via the intermediate stage of cartilage to bone, develops in islands. The main portion of any bone—the body—or its diaphysis, may be formed from one or more of these islands, described as "primary centers of ossification." They develop at various times during the latter months of fetal life and even during infancy. The epiphyses and appendages, such as tubercles and tuberosities, develop from additional centers of ossification, described as "secondary centers." Some of these develop as late as puberty or even adolescence.

In the earlier stages of this metaplasia into bone, there occurs a temporary deposition of calcium at the periphery of the growing island. As the border of calcium deposition advances, there develops behind it a rearrangement of the matrix and inorganic elements into actual bone. The first deposition is described as the "zone of temporary calcification." Normally, the width dimension of this zone is practically microscopic. However, in conditions such as some of the

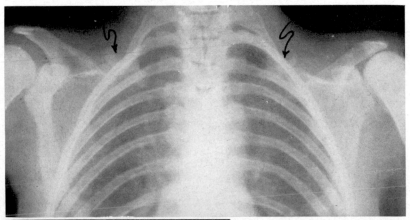

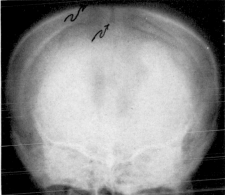

Fig. 30 (top).—Dysostosis of clavicles, likely due to deficient development of mesenchymal cords. Note miniature development of clavicles bilaterally. Associated dysostosis of cranial bones is common **(Fig. 31, middle). Fig. 32 (bottom).**—Pseudojoints, midclavicular region, probably due to "mesenchymal articulation"—joint action during mesenchymal rod formation.

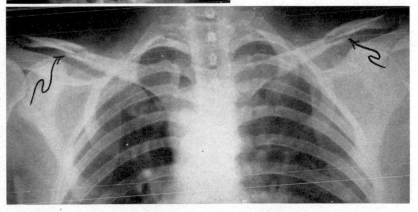

osteochondropathies, this zone may be of conspicuous width owing to delay in the final structural rearrangement. Except for the compact structures of the cortexes, true bone may be identified grossly by the arrangement of the inorganic constituents in a pattern featured by concentrations along lines of stress. These concentrations are described as "trabeculations."

Osteochondropathic derangements can be expected to occur particularly during the periods of transition from cartilage to calcification and from calcification to ossification. The age period differs for each region. The acute stage of a juvenile osteochondropathy involving any one primary center of ossification should be sought at a particular age, whereas similar changes concerned with the epiphyses or appendages—the secondary centers of ossification for one or another bone—are likely to be found at another particular age. It is important to correlate growth activity of any one region with diagnostic evaluations of roentgenographic evidence.

The articular cartilage, even though of the same type of cartilage (i.e., hyaline cartilage) as the temporary cartilage concerned with the development of bone, shows no tendency, normally, to become ossified. This same remarkable phenomenon pertains to disk cartilages. Such cartilages are therefore described as *permanent* or *adult cartilages*. They are devoid of vascular beds. They must receive their nourishment by osmosis from the vascular bed of the epiphyses and from secretions from the synovial membranes.

Normally, the vascular bed of the epiphysis extends by way of arcuate terminal vessels only to the dense osseous structure of the osseous articular cortexes. Under conditions of hypervascularity, such as might be stimulated when there is an infection in the joint or when trauma has been incurred with resultant fibrillation or fragmentation of a portion of the articular cartilage, there may result absorption of the dense structure of these cortexes, extension of the terminal vessels into these regions and thereafter calcification of the adult cartilages and, possibly, even ossifications, particularly at the joint margins. It appears that when the vascular bed is advanced in this manner, the otherwise permanent cartilage becomes calcified and eventually ossified, producing lippings, spur formations and similar abnormalities.

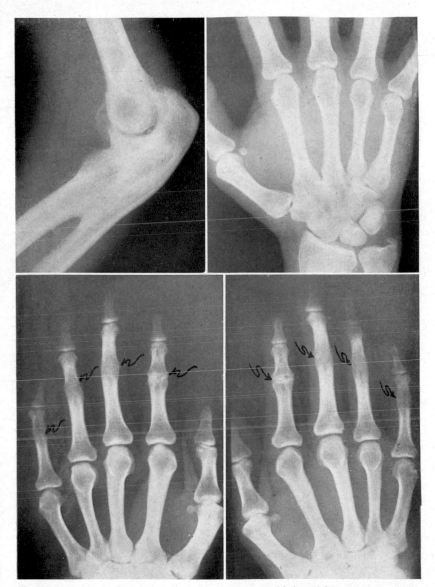

Fig. 33 (left above).—Synarthrosis of radius and ulna, result of failure of distinct formation of mesenchymal cords and joint separation. **Fig. 34 (right above).**—Synarthrosis of carpals and second,
third and fourth metacarpal joints. Note normal joint formation between semilunar and triquetral and
between these and the carpal mass; also malformation of ulnar styloid. Such malformations must not be
mistaken for ankylosis such as that from infectious arthritis. **Figs. 35 and 36 (below).**—Congenital
absence of interphalangeal joints (hereditary multiple ankylosing arthropathy). Note partial development
of proximal interphalangeal joint of index fingers but lack of such in third to fifth digits bilaterally.

As previously stated, the synovial membrane (synovialis) is fused into the circumference of articular cartilages. Although in fetal life it actually extends over the surfaces of these cartilages, it is normally obliterated as a distinct lining, particularly on the weight-bearing surfaces of the cartilages. In certain conditions such as atrophic arthritis and low grade infectious arthritis, or even following trauma (unless continuous activity is imposed), proliferation of the synovium may be so extensive as to produce a pannus or sheet coverage of the cartilaginous surfaces. This reaction has prompted the description "proliferative arthritis."

Strangely enough, although the synovial membrane does not normally cover the articular cartilages in the adult, it does invest certain interarticular cartilages such as those of the knee and temporomandibular joints. The menisci, or disks, of these joints are attached to the capsule by virtue of the synovial covering of their articular surfaces; in addition, they are intimately joined to the more tendinous strands of the outer joint sheath.

The synovial membrane must be recognized as simply the inner layer of the joint capsule. It is the secreting layer, serving both to lubricate the joint and to assist in providing nourishment to the articular and intra-articular cartilages. It may develop redundant folds, particularly along the edges of the articular cortexes. It may contain large fat collections as, for instance, in regions which would otherwise be unoccupied space, such as the intercondylar fossae. Such regions may appear roentgenographically as areas of increased density because fat is so ray transparent. Occasionally clusters of cartilaginous cells develop in these folds of synovia and may become ossified, resulting in "osteochondromatosis." They may become detached and thereby account for one source of *joint mice*. The folds themselves can be considered normal constituents of the joints. Particularly when pneumo-arthrography is performed, one must recognize them and avoid rash interpretations of "filling defects" or irregularities in the internal relief of the joint space.

Ligamentous structures may be located in the joint. They may thereby provide support in addition to that provided by the capsule, its ligamentous structures and the more peripherally located auxiliary ligaments and tendons. An example of an intra-articular liga-

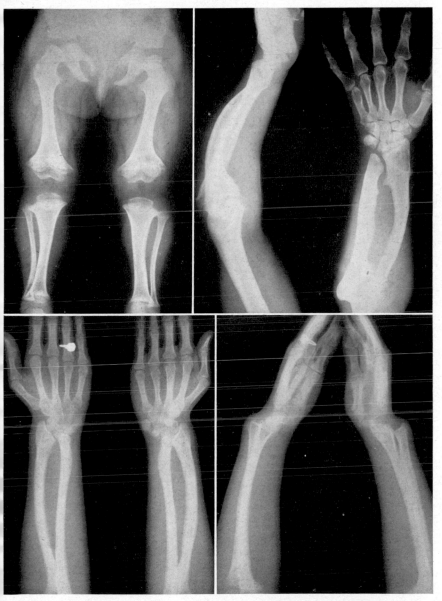

Dyschondroplasia. Several types of abnormal metaplasia of cartilage may occur. **Fig. 37 (left above).—** Such a case, misinterpreted as rickets. **Fig. 38 (right above).—**Madelung's deformity in patient with cartilaginous malformations throughout the body. Note relative shortness of forearm, double curvature of radius, interosseous excrescences, short ulna (due to premature fusion of its epiphysis); triangular arrangement of carpals. **Figs. 39 and 40 (below).—**Madelung's deformity, bilateral. Note lateral bowing of radii, widening of interosseous spacing, triangular arrangement of carpals, dorsal deviation of styloid extremity of ulna, dorsal bowing of radius.

ment is the ligamentum teres in the hip joint. Roentgenologically, it is important to consider the condition of such a structure.

In short, the character of the physiologic function of a particular joint is primarily responsible for its anatomic development. It determines whether or not the spacing between two bones will be composed merely of fibrous tissues or whether fibrous tissues and cartilages with a true joint space, or these with intra-articular cartilages, will be developed. Pathologic conditions cause destruction of certain constituents or rearrangements of others. All of these aspects: physiologic, embryologic, anatomic and pathologic, must be considered in analyzing the roentgenographic evidence.

BIBLIOGRAPHY

Brailsford, J. F.: Dystrophies of Skeleton, Brit. J. Radiol. 8:533–569, 1935.

Bromer, R. S.: Osteogenesis Imperfecta, Am. J. Roentgenol. 30:631–640, 1933.

Dannenberg, M.; Anton, J. I., and Spiegel, M. B.: Madelung's Deformity; Consideration of Its Roentgenological Diagnostic Criteria, Am. J. Roentgenol. 42:671–676, 1939.

Gray, H.: Anatomy of the Human Body (21st ed., rev. by W. H. Lewis; Philadelphia: Lea & Febiger, 1924).

Hill, L. L., Jr.: Congenital Abnormalities—Phocomelus and Congenital Absence of Radius, Surg., Gynec. & Obst. 65:475–479, 1937.

Pirie, A. H.: Marble Bones, Am. J. Roentgenol. 30:618–620, 1933.

Scaglietti, O.: Obstetrical Shoulder Trauma, Surg., Gynec. & Obst. 66:868–877, 1938.

Wilcox, L. F.: Osteopoikilosis, Am. J. Roentgenol. 30:615–617, 1933.

Zadek, I.: Congenital Coxa Vara, Arch. Surg. 30:62–102, 1935.

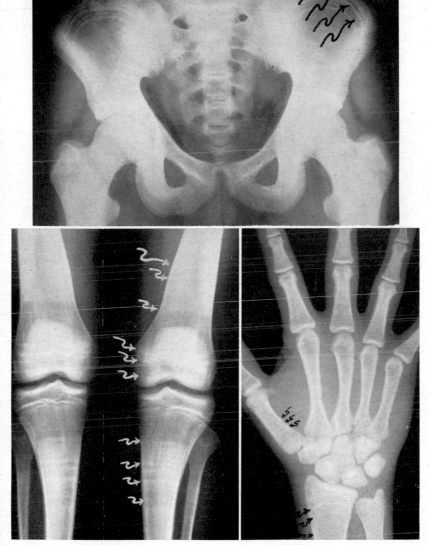

Figs. 41–43.—Growth lines *(Querstreifen)* may indicate periodic abnormalities in transition of cartilaginous skeleton into bone. They may be of such degree as to produce a brittle type of bone, as found in marble bone disease (Albers-Schönberg's disease), and cause bendings, fractures, deformities and malfunction of joints.

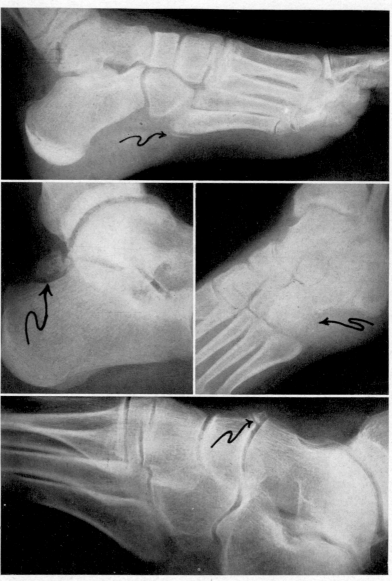

Ununited ossification centers. In the adult, they are described as ossicles. They must not be misinterpreted as fractures near or into the joint. **Fig. 44 (top).**—Note distal epiphyses of tibia and fibula, apophysis of the calcaneus, location of epiphyses of first metatarsal and all the phalanges at the proximal extremities and epiphyses of other metatarsals at the distal extremities. *Arrow points to epiphysis of base of fifth metatarsal, an os vesalianum.* **Fig. 45 (left center).**—*Arrow points to os trigonum, which might readily be misinterpreted as fracture of tuberosity of the astragalus.* **Figure 46 (right center)** shows the os peroneum and **Figure 47 (bottom)** the os epinaviculare.

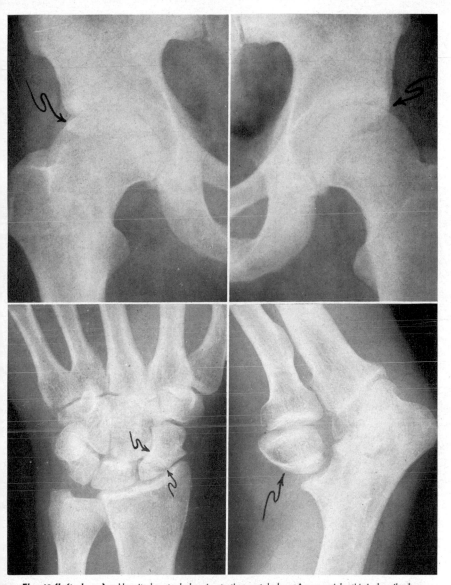

Fig. 48 (left above).—Ununited center belonging to the acetabulum. As an ossicle, this is described as an os acetabulum. It must not be misinterpreted as joint mouse. **Fig. 49 (right above).**—Same case. Partially attached secondary center—opposite side. **Fig. 50 (left below).**—Bipartite navicular, due to failure of union of two centers of ossification; distinguished from fracture by smooth, even borders, in contrast to sharp irregular borders of fractures. When present, it is likely to be bilateral. **Fig. 51 (right below).**—Joint formation around ununited secondary center of ossification—the radial condyle of the humerus.

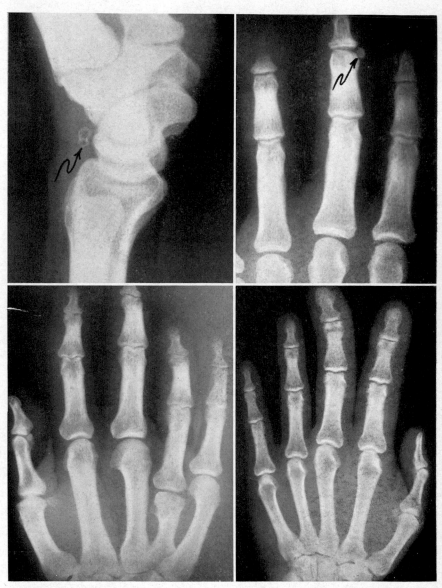

Fig. 52 (left above).—Ununited secondary center of ossification—os epilunatum. **Fig. 53 (right above).**—Ossicle belonging to head of the second phalanx, middle finger. **Fig. 54 (left below).**—Stunted growth of metacarpal due to failure of epiphyseal development. **Fig. 55 (right below).**—Macrodactyly, in contrast to foregoing condition, is an overgrowth of the digits (index and middle finger of left hand), produced when arteriovenous aneurysm or hemangioma causes oversupply of blood during growth period.

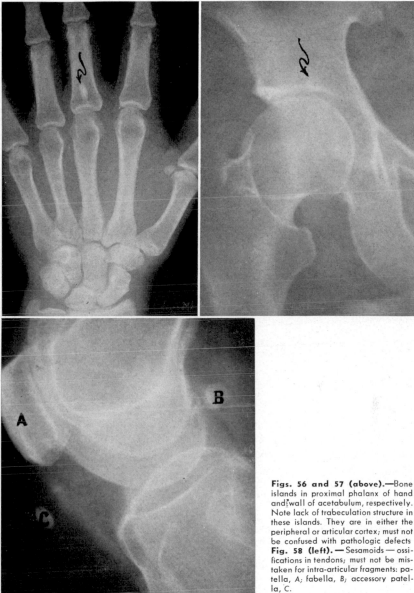

Figs. 56 and 57 (above).—Bone islands in proximal phalanx of hand and wall of acetabulum, respectively. Note lack of trabeculation structure in these islands. They are in either the peripheral or articular cortex; must not be confused with pathologic defects

Fig. 58 (left). — Sesamoids — ossifications in tendons; must not be mistaken for intra-articular fragments: patella, *A*; fabella, *B*; accessory patella, *C*.

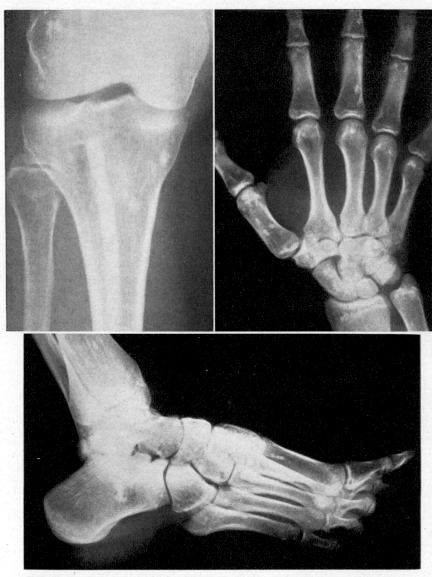

Figs. 59–61.—Multiple bone islands, including striations of nontrabeculated bone. When these condensations occur in size or numbers as found here, the condition is described as osteopoikilosis (osteopathia condensans disseminata; osteopecilia; osteopetrosis; etc.). They must not be interpreted as being of pathologic significance.

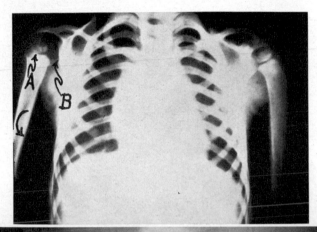

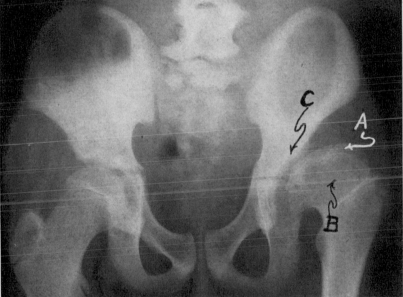

Congenital dislocations, also described as obstetrical joints. Abnormal function, likely based on deficient ligamentous support, seems responsible for subnormal developments and malformations. In **Figure 62 (above),** note the position of abduction and rotation of right humerus; delayed ossification of its capital epiphysis, A; elevation and rotation of the scapula; delayed ossification of head of scapula, B. In **Figure 63 (below),** note delayed and subnormal development of capital epiphysis, A; its flattening, and broadening of the neck, B; flattening of the acetabulum, C. Stereoscopy should establish malpositions, though often the relations are indefinite because of unossified cartilage. Later, these conditions may be mistaken for osteochondropathy.

Syphilitic Osteochondropathy

SYNONYMS: Congenital syphilis, hereditary syphilis, heredosyphilis (more specifically applied to group in which the disease is acquired during earlier months of fetal life), syphilitic dystrophy.

ROENTGEN CRITERIA

EARLY STAGES

Soft Tissues: Slight to moderate swelling.

Regional bones: Widening of zone of ossification (2–4 mm.), "the truly nutritional defect" (Vogt); irregular serration of its metaphysis; duplication of lines of ossification (zone of decreased tissue density —granulation tissue outside permanent ossification and between it and new line of temporary calcification—seen at extremities of diaphyses as well as at the periphery of epiphyses, if the latter are ossified); possibly, patchy rarefactions disseminated through the diaphysis or tables of the skull (vs. widespread deossification, as in rickets); disintegration erosions, angles of diaphyseal extremities (a most reliable criterion), especially inner aspects, upper extremities of tibiae (Wimberger's sign); possibly, periosteal expansions (as in dactylitis) or thickening and scalloping proliferation; possibly, fragmentations or infractions of diaphyseal extremities; possibly, luxation of epiphyses; rarely, widespread bone destruction and bone production—osteoporosis hypertrophica of Pick.

Articular cortexes: Likely, normal.

Joint space: Possibly, expanded.

LATER STAGES

Soft tissues: Atrophy.

Regional bones: Reossifications with conspicuous sclerosis of trabeculation pattern—condensing osteitis (i.e., Parrot's nodes, in skull); likely, temporary deformities (sites of infractions); likely, temporary or prolonged thickening of cortexes.

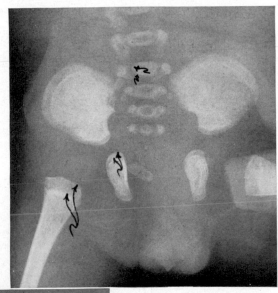

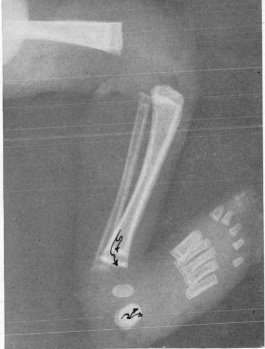

Figs. 64 and 65.—Findings in new-born. *Arrows* point to double lines of condensation, indicating zones of ossification and calcification with intervening pathology. Note multiplicity and bilaterality of involvement, with abnormalities at extremities of diaphyses and peripheries of epiphyses.

months, with increased cell count; albumin and globulin and, possibly, evidence obtained from the colloidal gold curve.

Biopsy: Finding of Treponema pallidum in maternal placenta or in tissues of the child (e.g., exudate from skin eruption, etc.).

CLINICAL COURSE: Favorable response to antisyphilitic treatment with involution of bone-cartilage lesions though positive serology persists for months or years.

BIBLIOGRAPHY

CAFFEY, J.: Syphilis of Skeleton in Early Infancy, Am. J. Roentgenol. 42:637–655, 1939.

EVANS, W. A.: Syphilis of Bones in Infancy, J. A. M. A. 115:197–200, 1940.

JEANS, P. C.: Congenital Syphilis, in Brennemann's Practice of Pediatrics (Hagerstown, Md.: W. F. Prior Company, Inc., 1942), Vol. II, ch. xxvi, pp. 6–52.

McCORD, J. R.: Osteochondritis in Stillborn, Am. J. Obst. & Gynec. 42:667–676, 1941.

McDONALD, D. H., AND SELLERS, E. D.: Pulmonary and Bony Changes in Congenital Syphilis, Texas State J. Med. 35:838–840, 1940.

McLEAN, S.: Roentgenographic and Pathologic Aspects of Congenital Osseous Syphilis, Am. J. Dis. Child. 41:130–152, 1931.

PARK, E. A., AND JACKSON, D. A.: Irregular Extensions of End of Shaft in X-Ray Photograph in Congenital Syphilis, with Pertinent Observations, J. Pediat. 13:748–759, 1938.

PARROT, J. M. J.: Maladies des enfants la syphilis hérédétaire et le rachitis ouvrage publié par les soins du Dr. Proisier [Diseases of infants; hereditary syphilis and rickets] (Paris: G. Masson, 1866), Vol. XXII, ch. viii, p. 321.

PENDERGRASS, E. P., AND BROMER, R. S.: Congenital Bone Syphilis, Am. J. Roentgenol. 22:1–21, 1929.

SARNAT, B. G.; SCHOUR, I., AND HEUPEL, R.: Roentgenographic Diagnosis of Congenital Syphilis in Unerupted Permanent Teeth, J. A. M. A. 116:2745–2747, 1941.

VOGT, E. C.: Value of Roentgenography in Diagnosis of Congenital Syphilis; Infants Considered, Am. J. Roentgenol. 26:96–101, 1931.

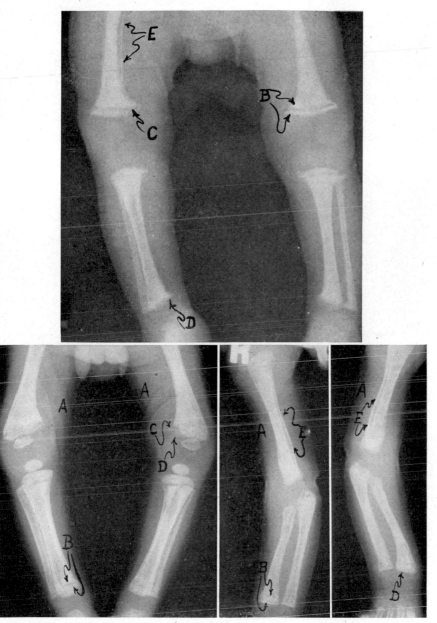

Figs. 69-72.—Late stage, showing: atrophy of soft tissues, *A;* duplication of zone of ossification, *B;* disintegration erosions, angles of diaphyses, *C;* infractions, *D;* periosteal condensations, *E.* General state of ossification is good.

Joint space: Likely, normal.
Deformities: Valgus or varus, knees and/or ankles.

CORROBORATIVE ROENTGEN CRITERIA: Sites of conspicuous pathology vary according to location of the greatest growth
activity for the particular age: i.e., first year, cranium or thorax;
second or third year, diaphyseal extremities of ulna, tibia or femur
and delay in closure of fontanels and union of secondary centers of
ossification; after puberty, metaphyseal reserve sites, cortexes and
finally the epiphyses—with progressive deossification.

INCIDENCE:
Age: Active stages, usually between third month and third year;
thereafter, likely at the age of puberty.
Sex: Irrelevant.
Geography: Temperate climates, particularly in western Europe,
Canada and the United States.
Habitat: More frequently found among poor city dwellers.
Race: Dark-skinned peoples especially susceptible (Negroes,
Italians).
Latitude: Mild or absent in tropics; highest incidence in temperate
zones; rare in frigid zone because of high fat diet.

HISTORY: Frequently, premature birth; restlessness, irritability,
sweating of the head, gastro-intestinal upsets and respiratory infections; likely, delay in sitting or standing.

PHYSICAL FINDINGS: Likely, an anemic appearing, inactive
child with apprehensive facies. Possibly, hot-cross bun configuration
of skull; Harrison groove configuration of thorax; possibly, deformities of extremities such as genu valgus or varus; prominent abdomen;
flaccid muscles; possibly, tenderness of bony prominences—skull,
knees and elbows.

LABORATORY FINDINGS
Blood: Calcium, likely, less than 9 mg. per 100 cc.; inorganic
phosphorus, likely, as low as 1.5 mg. per 100 cc. or less (calcium-
phosphorus product below 30); red cells and hemoglobin, likely,
reduced.

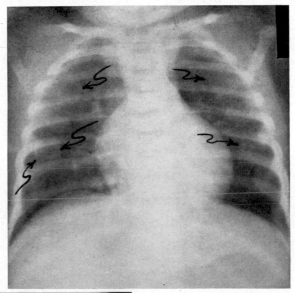

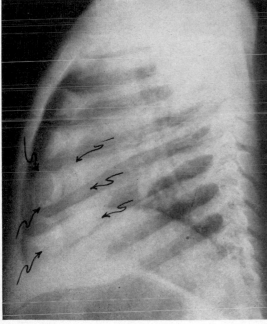

Figs. 76 and 77.—Active rickets, presenting vague outlines of costochondral junctions and flaring of osseous extremities.

CLINICAL COURSE: Rapid improvement after administration of vitamin D and inorganic elements; reossifications in two to four weeks.

BIBLIOGRAPHY

Boyd, J. D., AND Stearns, G.: Late Rickets Resembling Fanconi Syndrome, Am. J. Dis. Child. 61:1012–1022, 1941.

Caffey, J.: Lead Poisoning Associated with Active Rickets; Report of Case with Absence of Lead Lines in Skeleton, Am. J. Dis. Child. 55:798–806, 1938.

Chiari, O.: Beitrag zur Röntgendiagnose der floriden Rachitis [Roentgen diagnosis of fulminating rickets], Monatschr. f. Kinderh. 68:263–268, 1937.

Clements, F. W.: Rickets in Infants Aged under One Year; Incidence in Australian Community and Consideration of Ætiological Factors, M. J. Australia 1:336–346, 1942.

Cooley, T. B., AND Reynolds, L.: Interpretation of X-Ray Films in Diagnosis of Rickets, J. Pediat. 10:743–747, 1937.

Eliot, M. M., AND Park, E. A.: Rickets, in Brennemann's Practice of Pediatrics, (Hagerstown, Md.: W. F. Prior Company, Inc., 1942), Vol. I, ch. xxxvi, pp. 1–110.

Gezelius, G.: Über Rachitis bei Kindern nomadisierender Lappen [Concerning rickets among children of nomadic Lapps], Acta paediat. 26:184–193, 1939.

Giordano, J. J.: Raquitismo di la primera infancia [Rickets in infants in province of San Juan], Semana méd. 1:460–466, 1939.

Graser, E.: Rachitishäufigkeit unter Spätwinterkindern einer Grosstadt [Frequency of rickets in city children born in late winter], Ztschr. f. Kinderh. 61:520–532, 1939.

Hess, A. F.: Rickets Including Osteomalacia and Tetany (Philadelphia: Lea & Febiger, 1929).

Klotz, M.: Überlegungen zur Frage der Rachitis hepatica [Concerning a case of hepatic rickets], Monatschr. f. Kinderh. 79:39–42, 1939.

Knutsson, F.: Die röntgenologische Frühdiagnose der Rachitis [Early roentgen diagnoses of rickets], Acta paediat. 24:403–421, 1939.

Levesque, J.: Deux problèmes touchant le rachitisme: rachitisme rénal et rachitisme tardif [Two problems concerning rickets: renal rickets and late rickets], Bull. méd., Paris 53:55–60, 1939.

Lindblom, K.: Early Roentgen Signs in Rickets, Acta paediat. 25:170–180, 1939.

Park, E. A.: Observations on Pathology of Rickets with Particular Reference to Changes at Cartilage-Shaft Junctions of Growing Bones; Harvey Lecture, Bull. New York Acad. Med. 15:495–543, 1939.

Parsons, L. G.: Bone Changes Occurring in Renal and Coeliac Infantilism and Their Relationship to Rickets; Coeliac Rickets, Arch. Dis. Child. 2:198–211, 1927.

Price, N. L., AND Davie, T. B.: Renal Rickets, Brit. J. Surg. 24:548–569, 1937.

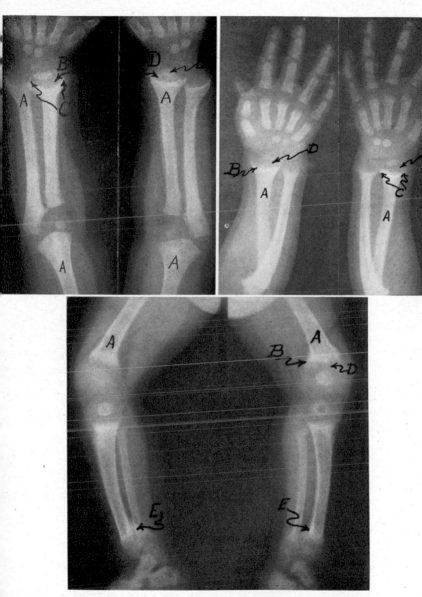

Figs. 78–80.—Active rickets. Widespread deossifications, *A;* widening of zones of calcification, *B;* saucerization with longitudinal beakings of the metaphyses, *C;* diaphyseal-epiphyseal spacings *D;* diaphyseal fractures, *E.*

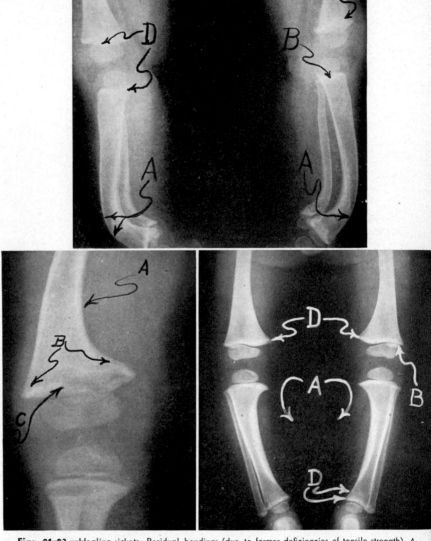

Figs. 81-83.—Healing rickets. Residual bendings (due to former deficiencies of tensile strength), A; residua of saucerization, B; healing diaphyseal fragmentation, C; condensations at zones of ossification (future growth lines), D.

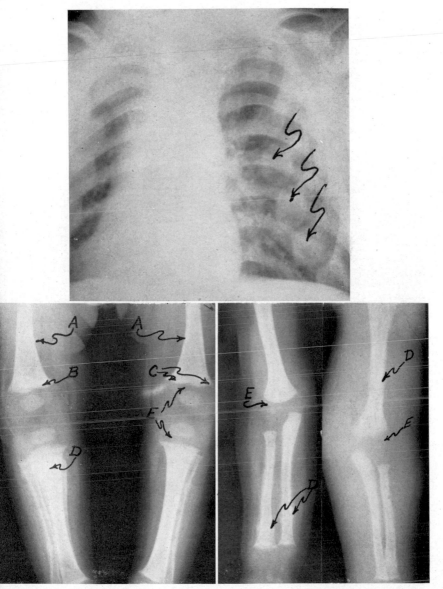

Healing stages. **Figure 84 (above)** shows costochondral beading, now conspicuous because of ossification of the tufted rib extremities. **Figs. 85 and 86 (below).**—Residual bending, A; widened zones of ossification, B; residual flaring of diaphyseal extremities, C; evidence of old fracture, D; greater than normal epiphyseal-diaphyseal spacing, E. In Figure 85, note evidence of combined scurvy—the scurvy zone in proximal extremities of tibiae and subperiosteal calcification.

to conspicuous healing, zone or limit of normal ossification vs. Fraenkel's white line and Wimberger's line); likely, residual transverse condensations (growth lines).

Articular cortexes: Normal.

Joint space: Normal.

CORROBORATIVE ROENTGEN CRITERIA: Findings most conspicuous in weight-bearing regions (diaphyseal extremities of the femur, tibia and their epiphyses); possibly, knoblike densities, costochondral junctions—indicative of hemorrhage.

INCIDENCE

Age: 3 months to 4 years; conspicuous osseous changes rare during later years.

Sex: Irrelevant.

Nutrition: Disease seldom or never found in breast-fed children (vitamin destroyed with pasteurization).

HISTORY: Irritability, anorexia, loss of weight, pain on motion, swelling, soreness and bleeding of gums and lack of fruit juices in diet.

PHYSICAL FINDINGS: Patient usually bedridden, guarding against movements of the extremities; facies apprehensive regarding handling. Usually, obvious underweight; likely, no evidence of toxicity, though temperature may be 100–101 F.; possibly, superficial ecchymoses (subcutaneous or submucous—in particular, regional to the teeth); likely, gums swollen; possibly, loss of one or more teeth (due to hemorrhage); possibly, exophthalmos; conjunctivas likely injected and possibly showing extravasations; costochondral and periarticular swellings may be prominent and the regions are likely to be tender on digital pressure. Muscular weakness may be noticeable, particularly on raising the head or extremities.

LABORATORY FINDINGS

Blood: Red cells—likely reduced to 3,500,000 or less; possibly, some nucleated; possibly, achromia, anisocytosis or polychromatophilia. Hemoglobin likely reduced to 70 per cent or less (color index normal). White cells—usually, some leukocytosis (to 21,000). with increase in polymorphonuclear neutrophils.

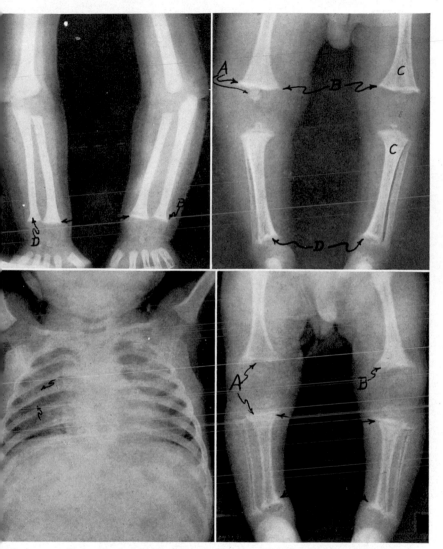

Early stages. **Figures 90 and 91 (above) and Figure 93 (right below)** show condensations, extremities of diaphyses (Fraenkel's white line) and peripheries of epiphyses (Wimberger's sign), A; metaphyseal spurs (Pelkan's spurs), B; deossifications and diaphyseal infractions, C; scurvy zone (*Trümmerfeldzone*), D. In the thorax **(Fig. 92, left below),** note sharp margination of costal beading (vs. poorly marginated tufting of active rickets).

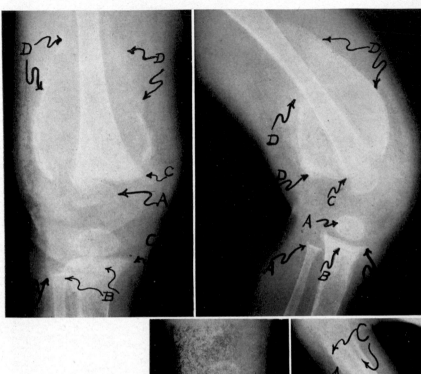

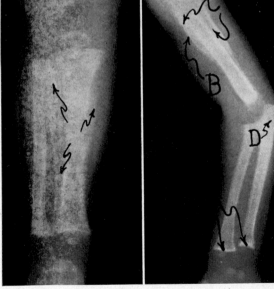

Figs. 98 and 99 (above).— Early healing stage. Condensation zones, extremities of diaphyses (Fraenkel's white line) and peripheries of epiphyses (Wimberger's sign), A; residual scurvy zone, B; metaphyseal spurs, C; periosteal elevations and subperiosteal calcifications, D. **Figs. 100 and 101 (right).—**Later stages. Condensations, extremities of diaphyses, A; periosteal elevations, B; actual subperiosteal reossification, C. Ground-glass appearance of the active stage has been replaced by substantial ossification through the main portions of bones, D.

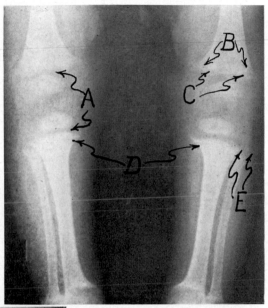

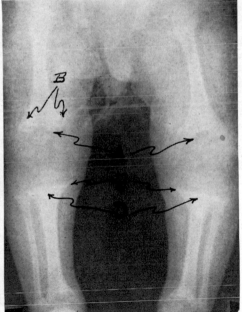

Figs. 102 and 103.—Combined rickets and scurvy. Epiphyseal-diaphyseal spacing, A; flaring of diaphyseal extremities, B; fraying of metaphyses, as found in rickets, C, scurvy zone, D; metaphyseal spurs; E—features of scurvy.

of acetabulum; likely, subcortical cystic dissolutions and condensations along metaphysis; likely, widening and shortening, and possibly bending, of femoral neck and diminution of normal angle between neck and shaft.

Articular cortexes: Likely, widening, flattening and irregularities; possibly, subarticular cystic dissolutions; possibly, eburnations; possibly, marginal spur formations.

Joint space: Likely, normal; possibly, slight reduction.

CORROBORATIVE ROENTGEN CRITERIA: Possibly, manifestations of remote rickets, other nutritional disturbances or endocrine disorder.

INCIDENCE

Age: Stage of greatest activity of growth of the epiphysis—usually between 3 and 10 years; residua throughout life.

Sex: Active males more frequently involved (six or more males to one female—Waldenström).

Bilaterality: Approximately 12 per cent of cases.

HISTORY: Possibly, remote history of trauma; possibly, rickets or localized infections; usually, insidious development of pain, aggravated by adduction and abduction; development of limp and limitation of hip movement; symptoms usually low grade and persisting 6–18 months.

PHYSICAL FINDINGS: Usually, healthy appearing child presenting no evidence of toxicity but manifestly guarding hip by flexing it; temperature, pulse and respiration normal. During active stages, elicitation of symptoms with adduction or abduction of the involved thigh. Likely, tenderness on digital pressure on groin; possibly, measurable shortening in dimensions of the involved lower extremity.

CLINICAL COURSE: Alleviation of symptoms with rest; physical well-being after six to nine months of inactivity and no specific treatment; likely, limp of slight to marked degree on resuming activities and, possibly, throughout life.

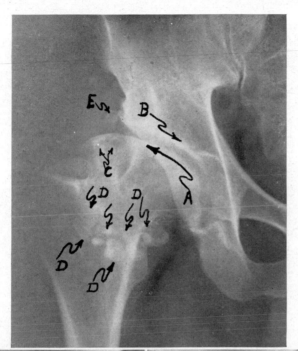

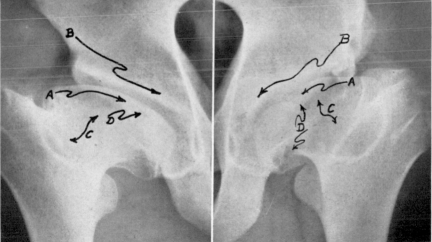

Residual changes. **Fig. 108 (above).**—Flattening of epiphysis, *A;* flattening and eburnation of acetabular cortex, *B;* subcortical cystic dissolutions, *C;* joint mice, resulting from fragmentations, *D;* fragmented spur, *E.* **Figs. 109 and 110 (below).**—Flattening of capital epiphysis, *A;* flattening, eburnation and spur formations of acetabular cortex, *B;* shortening of neck, *C;* subcortical cystic dissolution, *D.* Note reduction of angle between axis of neck and shaft.

BIBLIOGRAPHY

CALVÉ, J.: Sur une forme particulière de pseudo-coxalgie greffée sur des déformations caractéristiques de l'extrémité supérieure du fémur [Concerning a particular form of pseudo-coxalgia including characteristic deformities of the superior extremity of the femur], Rev. de chir. 30:54–84, 1910.

CAVANAUGH, L. A.; SHELTON, E. K., AND SUTHERLAND, R.: Metabolic Studies in Osteochondritis of the Capital Femoral Epiphysis, J. Bone & Joint Surg. 18:957–968, 1936.

DUNCAN, G. A.: Congenital Coxa Vara Occurring in Identical Twins, Am. J. Surg. 37:112–115, 1937.

GORALEWSKI, G., AND ENGEL, E.: Ein Beitrag zur Frage der Aetiologie der Osteochondritis coxae juvenilis—Perthes [Contribution to etiology of osteochondritis coxae juvenilis], Röntgenpraxis 4:745–747, 1932.

GÜTIG, K., AND HERZOG, A.: Die aseptische Schenkelhalsnekrose bei Jugendlichen. Osteochondritis juvenilis des Schenkelhalses [Aseptic necrosis of the neck of the femur in young persons. Osteochondritis juvenilis of the neck of the femur], Röntgenpraxis 4:504–513, 1932.

LANG, F. J.: Osteo-Arthritis Deformans Contrasted with Osteo-Arthritis Deformans Juvenilis, J. Bone & Joint Surg. 14:563–573, 1932.

LEGG, A. T.: Obscure Affection of the Hip Joint, Boston M. & S. J. 162:202–204, 1910.

ODEN, H. G.: Differentialdiagnose der Hüftgelenkstuberkulose und Perthesschen [Differential diagnosis between tuberculosis of the hip joint and Perthes' disease], Deutsches Tuberk.-Bl. 8:81–88, 1934.

PERTHES, G.: Über Osteochondritis deformans juvenilis [Concerning osteochondritis deformans juvenilis], Arch. f. klin. Chir. 101:779–807, 1913; also, Verhandl. d. deutsch. Gesellsch. f. Chir. 42:140–168, 1913.

WALDENSTRÖM, H.: The Definite Form of Coxa Plana, Acta radiol. 1:384–394, 1921–1922.

———: First Stages of Coxa Plana, J. Bone & Joint Surg. 20:559–566, 1938.

ZEMANSKY, A. P., JR.: Pathology and Pathogenesis of Legg-Calvé-Perthes' Disease (Osteochondritis Juvenilis Deformans Coxae), Am. J. Surg. 4:169–184, 1928.

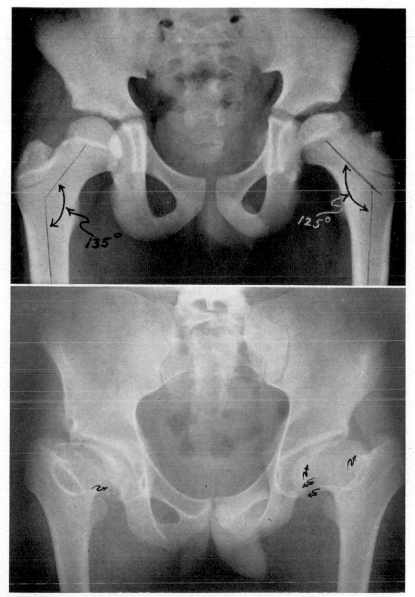

Residual changes following bone-cartilage damage. **Fig. 111 (above).**—Involvement on left, with shortening and expansion of neck and diminution of angle of neck with shaft. **Fig. 112 (below).**—Bilateral changes, including marked shortening of necks, "mushrooming" of heads with flattening of articular surfaces, both of heads of femora and of acetabula. *Arrows* point to cystic dissolutions.

Juvenile Osteochondropathy of the Tibial Tuberosity

SYNONYMS: Osgood-Schlatter's disease, apophysitis of the tibia.

ROENTGEN CRITERIA

EARLY STAGES

Soft tissues: Thickening of infrapatellar tendon; possibly, widespread edema with diffuse haziness around anterior aspects of the knee.

Regional bones: Delayed ossification of secondary centers concerned with the tuberosity; deossifications or actual rarefaction-erosions along borders of the ossifying tubercle, with deficient or delayed attachment and, possibly, anterior deviation in its position or a bending deformity; possibly, fragmentations; occasionally, extraneous calcifications projecting anteriorly or inferiorly into the infrapatellar tendon.

Articular cortexes: Normal.

Joint space: May be expanded.

LATER STAGES

Soft tissues: Likely, normal.

Regional bones: Possibly, lack of tibial tuberosity or deformation in its outline; likely, incomplete attachment, particularly at its lowermost extremity; possibly, fragmentations; usually, condensations along posterior border of attachment; frequently, isolated calcifications beyond normal limits of the bone (i.e., in the infrapatellar tendon).

Articular cortexes: Normal.

Joint space: Normal.

CORROBORATIVE ROENTGEN CRITERIA: Possibly, finding of old rickets, endocrine abnormalities or osteochondritis elsewhere.

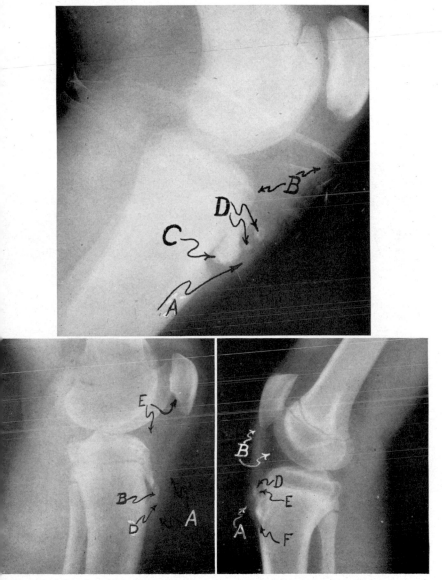

Figs. 113 (above) and 115 (right below).—Active stage. Widespread edema around tuberosity, *A;* thickening of infrapatellar tendon, *B;* anterior deviation of inferior extremity of tuberosity, *C;* fragmentations, *D;* deossification, *E;* deformity, *F.* **Fig. 114 (left below).**—Early subacute stage. Thickening of infrapatellar ligament, *A;* inhibited ossification, *B,* and deformity of tubercle; calcification in infrapatellar tendon, *D;* slight expansion of joint space ,*E.*

BRAILSFORD, J. F.: Osteochondritis, Brit. J. Radiol. 8:87–134, 1935.

BUCHMAN, J.: Résumé of Osteochondritides, Surg., Gynec. & Obst. 49:447–453, 1929.

————: Osteochondritis of Internal Cuneiform, J. Bone & Joint Surg. 15:225–232, 1933.

BURMAN, M. S.: Epiphysitis of Proximal or Pseudometatarsal Epiphyses of Foot, J. Bone & Joint Surg. 15:538–540, 1933.

————, AND LAPIDUS, P. W.: Unusual Appearance of Accessory Scaphoid and Styloid Epiphysis of Fifth Metatarsal, J. Bone & Joint Surg. 12:160–164, 1930.

CHRISTIE, A. C.: Osteochondritis or Epiphysitis, J. A. M. A. 87:291–295, 1926.

FREIBERG, A. H.: Infraction of Second Metatarsal Bone; A Typical Injury, Surg., Gynec. & Obst. 19:191–193, 1914.

GILLIES, C. L.: Kienböck's Disease of Semilunar Bone of Wrist, Am. J. Roentgenol. 30:1–7, 1933.

HARBIN, M.: Osteochondritis, Focal and Multiple, Am. J. Roentgenol. 29:763–765, 1933.

————, AND ZOLLINGER, R.: Osteochondritis of Growth Centers, Surg., Gynec. & Obst. 51:145–161, 1930.

KIENBÖCK, R.: Über traumatische Maladie des Mondbeins [On Traumatic Disease of the Semilunar], Fortschr. a. d. geb. d. Röntgenstrahlen 16:77, 1910.

KÖHLER, A.: History of Köhler's Disease, München. med. Wchnschr. 71:109, 1924.

LEWIN, P.: Osteochondritis Deformans Juvenilis of Shoulder Joint, J. Bone & Joint Surg. 9:456–457, 1927.

LIPSCOMB, P. R., AND CHATTERTON, C. C.: Osteochondritis Juvenilis of Acetabulum, J. Bone & Joint Surg. 24:372–381, 1942.

MARTIN, W. C., AND ROESLER, H.: Multiple Manifestations of Subchondral Necrosis (Osteochondropathia Juvenilis, Osteochondritis, Epiphysitis), Am. J. Roentgenol. 26:861–867, 1931.

MEYERDING, H. W., AND STUCK, W. G.: Painful Heels among Children (Apophysitis), J. A. M. A. 102:1658–1660, 1934.

PHEMISTER, D. B.; BRUNSCHWIG, A., AND DAY, L.: Streptococcal Infections of Epiphysis and Short Bones; Their Relation to Köhler's Disease of Tarsal Navicular, Legg-Perthes' Disease and Kienböck's Disease of Os Lunatum, J. A. M. A. 95:995–1002, 1930.

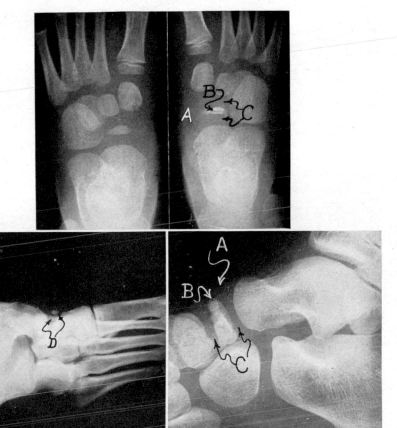

Figs. 128-130.—Osteochondropathy of the navicular (Köhler's disease of the tarsals). Swelling and slight edema of regional soft tissues, *A;* delayed development, disklike configuration, *B* (compare right and left sides, **Fig. 128, above);** sparing of interosseous spacing, *C.* **Figure 129 (left below)** shows residua of this condition—a rudimentary navicular fragmentation, *D.*

Physical activity: Usually strenuous.

Sites of involvement: In dissecans type, knee in approximately 85 per cent (usually, internal condyle of femur, lateral and posterior to insertion of the posterior cruciate ligament; rarely, external condyle or tibial aspect of the joint); elbow (usually, posterior aspect of capitellum); shoulder (head of humerus); hip (head of femur); wrist (radial aspect); ankle (tibial aspect) or talus; rarely, other joints or bones.

HISTORY: Trauma may be remotely associated; specific background for other than dissecans type—violent injury, radiation therapy, atmospheric pressure changes, etc. Likely, soreness or dull pain in joint, with weight-bearing or use, progressive increase in severity; possibly, local swelling; possibly, episodes of locking of the joint in position of flexion (i.e., following detachment of button or fragments); notable absence of fever or toxicity.

CLINICAL COURSE: Following removal, or fixation, of detached bone-cartilage island, probably no symptoms; possibly, later manifestation of static arthropathy.

BIBLIOGRAPHY

BELL, A. L. L.; EDSON, G. N., AND HORNICK, N.: Characteristic Bone and Joint Changes in Compressed-Air Workers, Radiology 38:698–707, 1942.

BENNETT, G. E.: Shoulder and Elbow Lesions of Professional Baseball Pitcher, J. A. M. A. 117:510–514, 1941.

CONWAY, F. M.: Osteochondritis Dissecans: Description of Stages of Condition and Its Probable Traumatic Etiology, Am. J. Surg. 38:691–699, 1937.

KING, D., AND RICHARDS, V.: Osteochondritis Dissecans of the Hip, J. Bone & Joint Surg. 22:327–348, 1940.

KÖNIG, F.: Lehrbuch der speciellen Chirurgie für Aerzte und Studierende [Text of Special Surgery for Physicians and Students], (Berlin: A. Hirschwald, 1889), p. 690.

ROMBOLD, C.: Osteochondritis Dissecans of the Patella, J. Bone & Joint Surg. 18:230–231, 1936.

WOLBACH, S. B., AND ALLISON, N.: Osteochondritis Dissecans, Arch. Surg. 16:1176–1186, 1928.

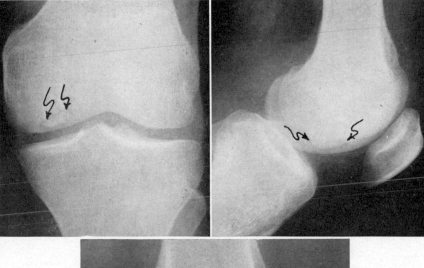

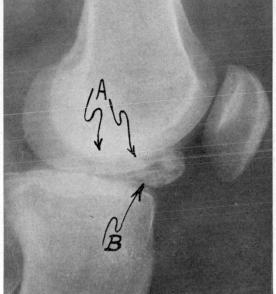

Most typical location for osteochondritic sequestration—the knee. Note particular location in internal condyle of femur, lateral to insertion of cruciate ligament. Initially, the sequestrated island is outlined by a double-contoured density *(arrows,* **Figs. 143 and 144, above).** Ultimately, this island may separate **(Fig. 145, below),** leaving an excavation in the articular cortex, *A,* becoming a migrating button of bone and cartilage (joint mouse), *B;* note its cystic dissolution.

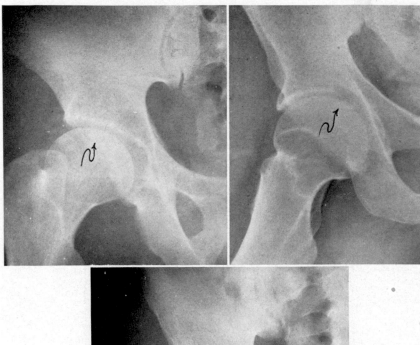

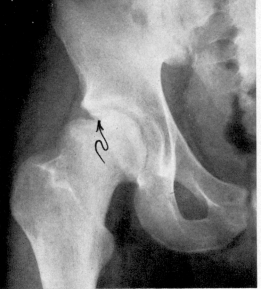

Figs. 146 and 147 (above).—Osteochondritic dissection in head of femur. Note double-contoured outline of sequestration.
Fig. 148 (below).—Similar case, later stage. Note evidence of absorption of button, roughening and cystic changes around border of concavity.

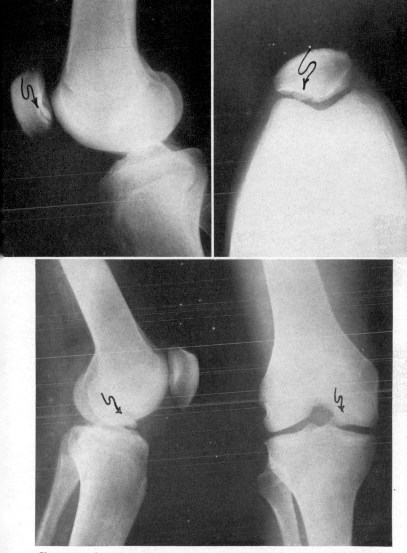

Figs. 149 and 150 (above).—Unusual osteochondritic dissection of cortex of the patella.
Fig. 151 (below).—Same case, opposite knee. This case emphasizes the multiplicity of involvement of this disease.

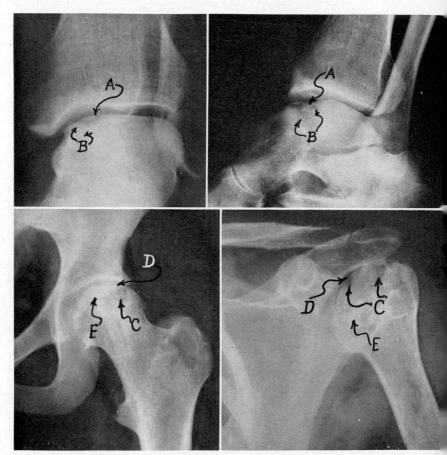

Figs. 152 and 153 (above).—Osteochondropathy, dissecans type, involving the ankle. Dissected bone-cartilage island, *A;* regional dissolution of bone in talus, *B.* **Figs. 154 and 155 (below).**— Similar manifestations of aseptic necrosis following severe fall. In both hip and shoulder, subcortical dissolutions, *C;* collapse of articular cortexes with flattening, *D;* osteosclerotic reaction, *E.* Such changes emphasize interrelationship of osteo-arthropathies and traumatic arthropathies. Note eventual changes of eburnations, marginal spurs, etc., as described in other sections.

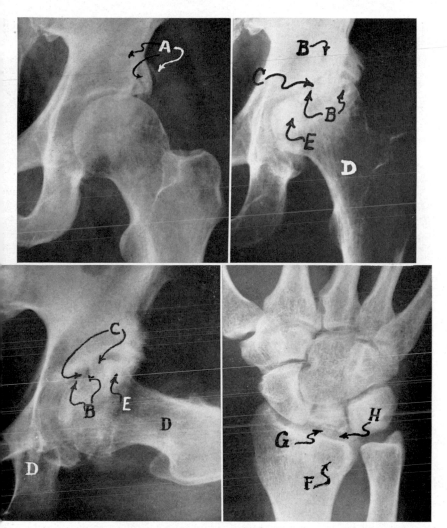

Bone-cartilage pathology based on aseptic necrosis of adult cartilage following trauma. **Fig. 156 (left above).**—Condition immediately after reduction of dislocation (in which disruption of the ligamentum teres undoubtedly occurred, with loss of its vascular supply); note fragmentation of superior rim of acetabulum, A. **Figs. 157 (right above) and 158 (left below).**—Findings 18 months later: cortical and subcortical cystic dissolutions, B; collapse of osseous articular cortex with flattening, C; extensive deossification (of disuse and, possibly, neurovascular), D; osteosclerosis, E. **Fig. 159 (right below).**—Similar changes in wrist of an adult—adult Kienböck's disease; note cystic dissolution in radius, F; fragmentation of proximal osseous articular cortex of lunate, G; obliteration of radius-lunate interosseous spacing, H (not found in juvenile type).

Osteo-Arthropathies: Traumatic*

SYNONYMS: Sprain, dislocation, traumatic synovial effusion; later—Leriche's atrophy, Sudeck's atrophy, tennis elbow, baseball shoulder, milk deliveryman's knee, hypertrophic arthritis.

ROENTGEN CRITERIA

EARLY STAGES

Soft tissues: Likely, *asymmetrical* edema with prominence of soft tissues and partial obliteration of fascial planes; possibly, partial detachment of periosteum at muscle origins or insertions.

Regional bones: Possibly, fractures; otherwise, normal osseous architecture.

Articular cortexes: Likely, normal; possibly, fracture.

Joint space: Likely, expansion with deviation of capsular outlines; possibly, increase in dimension between opposing osseous articular cortexes; possibly, asymmetry. Pneumo-arthrography may visualize fragmentations of articular cartilages or menisci or displacements of the latter.

LATER STAGES

Soft tissues: Likely, normal; possibly, some atrophy; possibly, residual edema (even though atrophy) with obliteration of fascial planes; possibly, containing calcifications.

Regional bones: Possibly, slight deossification; possibly, evidence of callus formation around fractures; likely, distortion of alinement.

Articular cortexes: Possibly, deossifications (may be conspicuous, with contrast in densities as compared with contiguous bone; possibly, thinning in vertical dimensions and irregularities in articular surfaces); possibly, eburnations with marginal spurs; possibly, dissolutions (necroses).

*This term should be used conservatively, since it is likely to imply blame and compensation rights.

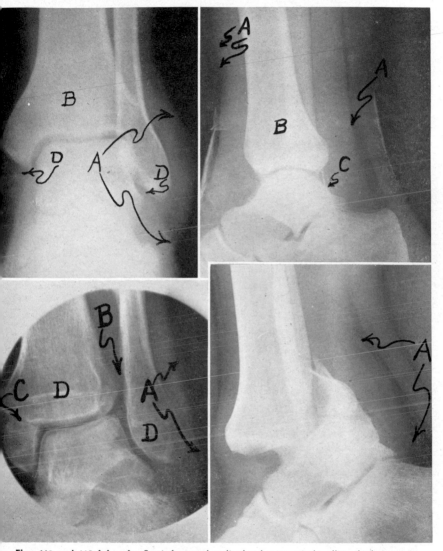

Figs. 168 and 169 (above).—Sprain-fracture. Localized and asymmetrical swelling of soft tissues, A; normal architecture of regional bones, B; slight periosteal detachment, C; expansion of joint space, D. **Fig. 170 (left below).**—Laceration of tibiofibular ligament. Swelling of soft tissues, A; increased space between tibia and fibula, B; fracture, C; beginning deossification (probably from disuse), D. **Fig. 171 (right below).**—Pott's fracture. Conspicuous localized swelling of soft tissues, A, with tendon deviation but no diffuse obliteration of posterior triangle. Compare localized swelling of trauma vs. periarticular edema of infection (see infectious arthritis).

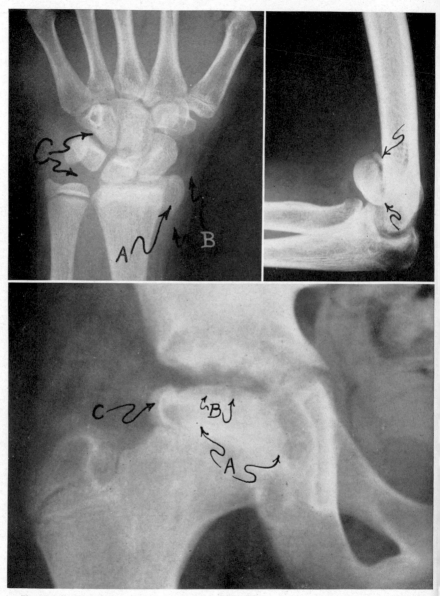

Fig. 176 (left above).—Epiphyseal separation. Considerable joint injury can be expected, with possible inhibition of growth and perhaps later, aseptic necrosis involving the epiphysis. Note malalinement, A; soft tissue edema, B; widening of joint space, C. **Fig. 177 (right above).**—Fragmentation of condyle, producing mechanical interference of joint function and loss of articular surfaces. **Fig. 178 (below).**—Hypertrophic changes in youth several years after epiphyseal separation. Note condensations, A; absorptions (avascular necrosis), B; metaphyseal spur, C.

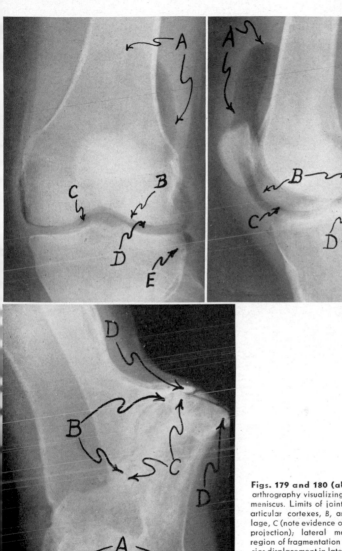

Figs. 179 and 180 (above).—Pneumo-arthrography visualizing deranged lateral meniscus. Limits of joint space, A, osseous articular cortexes, B, and articular cartilage, C (note evidence of erosion in lateral projection); lateral meniscus, D (note region of fragmentation in A-P and posterior displacement in lateral projection); air pocket beneath lateral fragment of meniscus, E. **Fig. 181 (left).**—Pseudojoint at site of old fracture of humerus. Elbow joint proper, A; false joint, B; eburnations along newly developed articular cortexes, C; marginal spurs, D.

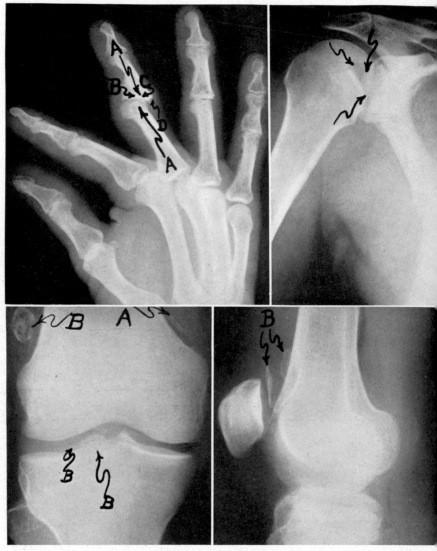

Fig. 190 (left above).—Chronic dislocation. Malalinement of bone, *A;* deformity of articular cortex, *B;* eburnation, *C;* marginal spur formations, *D.* **Fig. 191 (right above).**—Grooved defect in head of humerus; note smooth, rounded borders. History of severe injury, believed responsible for aseptic necrosis (the defect) and, as result, repeated dislocations. **Figs. 192 and 193 (below).**—Post-traumatic calcifications in internal collateral ligament, *A* (Pellegrini-Stieda's disease), and in synovial membrane, *B.*

Osteo-Arthropathies: Static

SYNONYMS: Progressive minimal traumatic arthritis, weight-bearing arthritis, postural arthritis, obesity arthritis, hypertrophic arthritis, osteo-arthritis, degenerative arthritis, dry arthritis.

ROENTGEN CRITERIA

EARLY STAGES

Soft tissues: Likely, excessive (fat and musculature).

Regional bones: Possibly, malalinements; likely, osseous architecture normal.

Articular cortexes: Likely, eburnations with marginal spur formations; possibly, flattening of articular surfaces.

Joint space: Likely, asymmetrical reduction of interosseous spacing.

LATER STAGES

Soft tissues: Likely, normal.

Regional bones: Likely, malalinements; likely, osseous architecture normal.

Articular cortexes: Eburnations with marginal spur formations.

Joint space: Asymmetrical narrowing of interosseous spacing; possibly, intra-articular fragments or calcifications.

CORROBORATIVE ROENTGEN CRITERIA: Involvement usually of weight-bearing joints; usually bilateral (except in mixed types).

INCIDENCE

Age: 25–50.

Sex: Males and females almost equally involved.

HISTORY: Prolonged period of excessive weight; interval attacks of "arthritis" in weight-bearing joints; possibly, episodes of definite infectious arthritis; possibly, episodes of locking or partial locking.

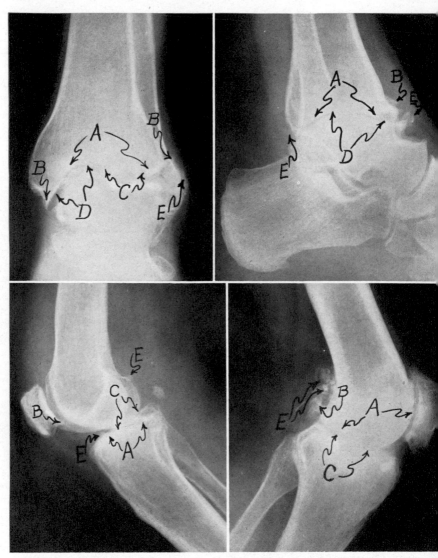

Figs. 205–208.—Mixed arthropathies; static changes superimposed on joints damaged by previous arthritic processes. Eburnations, *A;* marginal spurs, *B;* irregularities of osseous articular surfaces, *C;* reduction and asymmetry of interosseous spacing, *D;* intra-articular spurs and fragments, *E.*

Osteo-Arthropathies: Senescent

SYNONYMS: Hypertrophic arthritis, degenerative arthritis, osteo-arthritis, chondro-osseous arthritis, nonankylosing arthritis, climacteric arthritis, menopausal arthritis, dry arthritis, senile arthritis, type II arthritis—Ely, morbus coxae senilis, arthritis deformans—Virchow, Heberden's nodes.

ROENTGEN CRITERIA

EARLY STAGES

Soft tissues: Possibly, evidence of obesity; more than average (for age) muscular clothing; possibly, calcific streaking of arteries or phleboliths.

Regional bones: Depletion of metaphyseal reserve sites; narrowing of cortexes; coarsening of trabeculations.

Articular cortexes: Thinning; eburnations; marginal lipping; likely, irregularities of osseous articular surfaces (recession of one side compensated by prominence of opposite side).

Joint space: Possibly, asymmetrical with noticeable diminution of one or another portion.

LATER STAGES

Soft tissues: Likely, calcific streaking in vessels; possibly, phleboliths; likely, slight muscle atrophy with conspicuous and irregular fascial spaces.

Regional bones: Likely, deossification with depletion of metaphyseal shelving and, possibly, subcortical cysts.

Articular cortexes: Irregular eburnations; hypertrophic lipping and spur formations.

Joint space: Likely, reduced; possibly, containing joint mice (fragments of spurs, or calcified fatty degenerations in synovia); possibly, abnormalities in alinement because of partial subluxations. (Limitation of movement due to mechanical obstruction, i.e., Heberden's

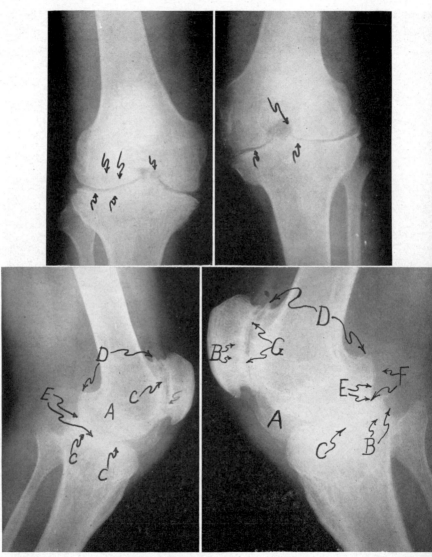

Late stage, in patient, 24. **Figs. 222 and 223 (above).**—Note weight-bearing joints; bilateral involvement; atrophy of soft tissues; eburnations and marginal spur formations. *Arrows* indicate areas of erosion. The patient's youth eliminates "hypertrophic arthritis" in the usual sense of the term. **Figs. 224 and 225 (below).**—Lateral projections, showing thinning of trabeculations, *A*; cystic dissolutions, *B*; eburnations, *C*; marginal spur formations, *D*; irregularities of articular surfaces, *E*; reduced joint spaces, *F*; cleavage line (fibrous ankylosis), *G*.

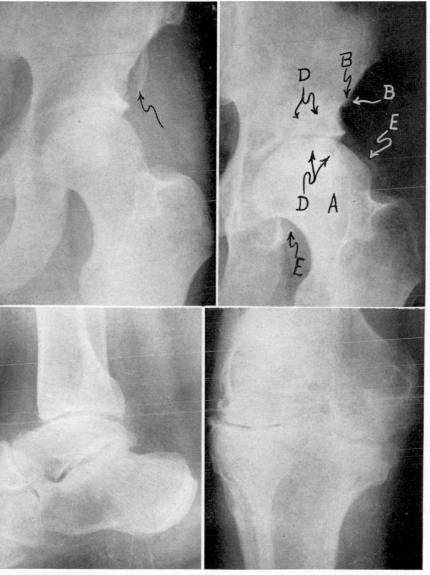

Changes in hemophiliac. **Fig. 226 (left above).**—Calcification of hemorrhage at site of muscle origin. **Fig. 227 (right above).**—Thinning of osseous trabeculations, *A*; spur formations at sites of muscle origin, *B*; thinning, and cystic erosion of articular cortexes, *D*; intra-articular calcification, *E*. **Figs. 228 and 229 (below).**—In both knees and ankles, flattening and irregularity of osseous articular surfaces; compression of bones, i.e., internal condyle of tibia and astragalus. Eburnations and spur formations might suggest "hypertrophic arthritis," which would not indicate etiology.

Neuro-Arthropathies: Simple

SYNONYMS: Motor nerve paralysis arthropathy, nerve atrophy of joints, sequela to acute poliomyelitis—Heine-Medin's disease.

ROENTGEN CRITERIA

EARLY STAGES

Soft tissues: Atrophy, possibly of selected muscle groups.
Regional bones: Widespread deossification.
Articular cortexes: Thinning.
Joint space: Normal.

LATER STAGES

Soft tissues: Atrophy, possibly of selected muscle groups; occasionally, para-articular calcifications.

Regional bones: Widespread deossifications; possibly, cystic dissolutions; possibly, diminished development or actual resorption of dimensions or configurations; occasionally, fractures with minimal strain.

Articular cortexes: Thinning; possibly, eburnations; possibly, marginal spur formations; irregularities and flattenings of articular surfaces.

Joint space: Likely, diminished; occasionally, subluxations.

CORROBORATIVE ROENTGEN CRITERIA: Involvement of a *series* of joints concerned with any one nerve trunk distribution; likely in one or both lower extremities or even an upper extremity.

INCIDENCE

Age: Acute symptoms most common between 2 and 5 (approximately 60 per cent); progressive decrease in incidence thereafter.

Sex: Males more frequently involved than females.

Season: Acute symptoms usually appear late in the spring, in the summer or early in the fall.

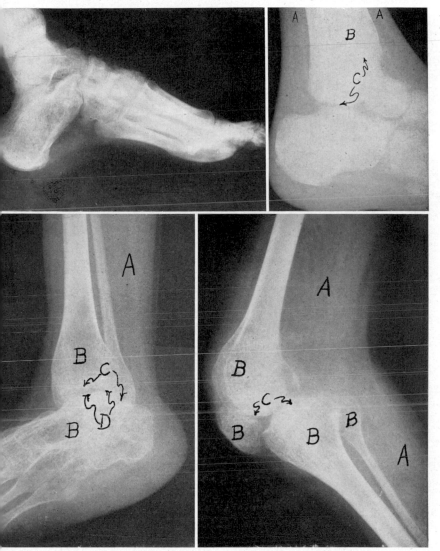

Pes cavus from imbalance of tendons following poliomyelitis. **Fig. 236 (left above).**—Note deossification and thinning of osseous articular cortexes. **Fig. 237 (right above).**—Atrophy of soft tissues, A; beginning deossification, B; slight irregularity and flattening of osseous articular surfaces, C. **Figs. 238 and 239 (below).**—Relatively early changes. Slight atrophy of muscles and tendons, A; deossification of regional bones, B; thinning of articular cortexes, C; irregularity and flattening of osseous articular surfaces, D.

HISTORY: Sudden onset of fever, malaise, gastro-intestinal disturbance; possibly, meningeal symptoms in a few days with headache, vomiting and stiffness of the neck and soon thereafter, flaccidity of one or several muscle groups.

PHYSICAL FINDINGS: In early stages, evidence of toxicity with fever 101-103 F.; possibly, stiffness of neck and resistance to flexion of spine; positive Koenig's and Brudzinski's signs; absent or diminished deep and superficial reflexes and, possibly, loss of sensation in one or another part. Later, there may be conspicuous muscle atrophy, flaccidity and abnormal mobility of one or another joint; possibly, deformities such as contractures or scoliotic changes; possibly, impaired growth.

LABORATORY FINDINGS

Blood: Red cells, slight anemia; white cells, moderate leukocytosis.

Spinal fluid: Clear to opalescent; increased protein and lymphocytes (during active stages).

BIBLIOGRAPHY

CORBIN, K. B., AND HINSEY, J. C.: Influence of Nervous System on Bones and Joints, Anat. Rec. 75:307–317, 1939.

FERGUSON, A. B.: Short Metatarsal Bones and Their Relationship to Poliomyelitis, J. Bone & Joint Surg. 15:98–100, 1933.

HASSIN, G. B.; BAKER, E. L., AND WAKEFIELD, H.: Roentgenographic Bone Changes in Second Case of Old Poliomyelitis, J. A. M. A. 85:267, 1925.

SCHEIN, A. J.: Orthopedic Aspects of Poliomyelitis, New York State J. Med. 37:1661–1667, 1937.

SHANDS, A. R., JR.: Neuropathies of Bones and Joints: Report of Case of Arthropathy of Ankle Due to Peripheral Nerve Lesion, Arch. Surg. 20:614–636, 1930.

WAREMBOURG, H., AND MERLEN: Poliomyélite antérieure aiguë et ostéo-arthrites multiples d'origine gonococcique [Acute anterior poliomyelitis and multiple osteo-arthritis], Echo méd. du Nord 5:404–409, 1936.

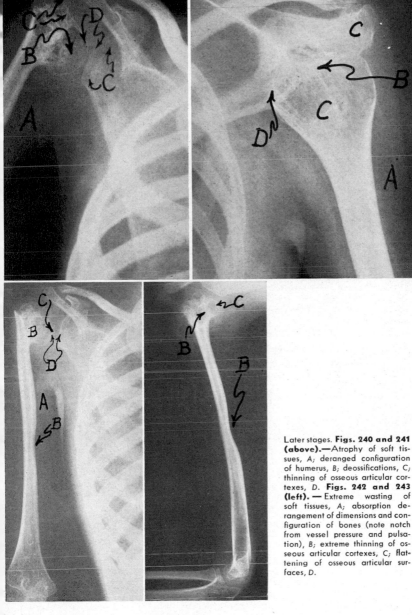

Later stages. **Figs. 240 and 241 (above).**—Atrophy of soft tissues, A; deranged configuration of humerus, B; deossifications, C; thinning of osseous articular cortexes, D. **Figs. 242 and 243 (left).** — Extreme wasting of soft tissues, A; absorption derangement of dimensions and configuration of bones (note notch from vessel pressure and pulsation), B; extreme thinning of osseous articular cortexes, C; flattening of osseous articular surfaces, D.

HISTORY: Variable, depending on basic disease: tabes dorsalis, leprosy, syringomyelia or posterior transverse myelitis.

PHYSICAL FINDINGS: Individual poorly nourished (due usually to physical limitations); temperature, pulse and respirations normal or only slightly elevated; likely, involved joints prominent and their use clumsy; no tenderness or pain on passive movement; loss of receptor sense to pinprick and similar tests over region involved; otherwise, findings variable depending on the particular condition.

LABORATORY FINDINGS: Variable, including positive serology (blood, synovial and spinal fluid), positive albumin and colloidal gold curve in the case of syphilis.

CLINICAL COURSE: Progressive destruction of osseous extremities with use.

BIBLIOGRAPHY

BARKER, L. F.: Neuropathic Arthropathies, Monographic Med. 4:116–117, 1920.
DUNCAN, J. H.: Neuropathic Arthritis, J.A.M.A. 79:1987–1989, 1922.
HODGSON, N., AND WHYTE, A. H.: Charcot's Disease of Ankle Joint, Newcastle M. J. 7:144–146, 1927.
KARASEFF, J.: Aspect radiographique des manifestations ostéo-articulaires dans la lèpre [Radiographic picture of bone and joint changes in leprosy], J. de radiol. et d'électrol. 20:373–382, 1936.
LEADER, S. A.: Charcot's Arthropathy of Both Ankles, Am. J. Roentgenol. 43:509–513, 1940.
MAJOR, R. H.: Charcot's Foot, J.A.M.A. 90:846, 1928.
MURDOCK, J. R., AND HUTTER, H. J.: Leprosy; Roentgenological Survey, Am. J. Roentgenol. 28:598–621, 1932.
VON PANNEWITZ, G.: Neuropathische Gelenkerkrankungen und ihre röntgenologische Frühdiagnose [Neuropathic articular disorders and their early diagnosis], Med. Klin. 32:1171–1174, 1936.
PHILIPS, H. B., AND ROSENHECK, C.: Neuroarthropathies; Consideration of Etiology and General Characteristics, J. A. M. A. 82:27–29, 1924.
SHANDS, A. R., JR.: Neuropathies of Bones and Joints; Report of Case of Arthropathy of Ankle Due to a Peripheral Nerve Lesion, Arch. Surg. 20:614–636, 1930.
STEINDLER, A.: Tabetic Arthropathies, J. A. M. A. 96:250–256, 1931.
WILE, U. J., AND BUTLER, M. G.: Critical Survey of Charcot's Arthropathy, J. A. M. A. 94:1053–1055, 1930.

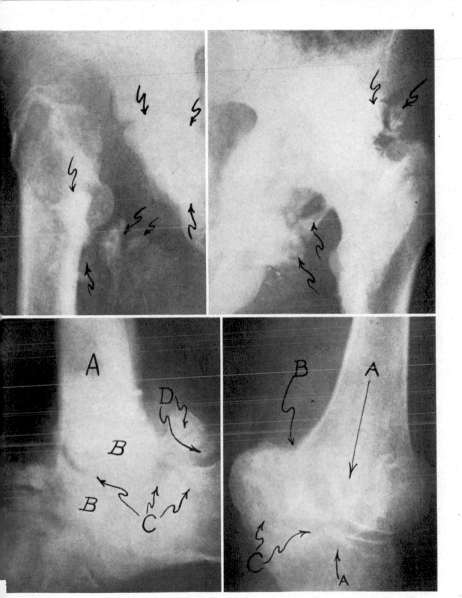

Separation of head of femur in **Figure 248 (left above)** and fragmentations in **Figure 249 (right above).** *Arrows* indicate detached fragments in joint space—prompting the expression "bag of bones." **Fig. 250 (left below).**—Tabetic ankle, late stage. Evidence of use regardless of severe destruction; substantial osseous architecture, *A*; condensations, *B*; impaction fragmentations, indicating continued punishment of bones, *C*; bone fragments in joint space, *D*. **Fig. 251 (right below).**—Changes in knee from transverse myelitis involving posterior tracts. Malalinement of bones, emphasizing postural traumatic factor, *A*; fragmentation of femoral condyle, *B*; destruction of osseous articular cortexes (and cartilage), *C*.

and clearing in three to seven days and other joints manifesting similar reactions before clearing of the first and also subsiding in a short time; possibly, intermittent episodes of such manifestations.

PHYSICAL FINDINGS: Possibly, manifest toxicity with anxious facies, definite fever, to 104 F.; usually, involved joints conspicuously swollen and red, with pitting edema but not tender. Subcutaneous nodules (Osler's nodes) may be palpated (especially to be sought along ulnar aspects of forearms, dorsa of hands, knees and on scalp). Thrill may be palpated over precordium; globular configuration in outline of cardiac dulness, and presystolic or systolic murmur likely in aortic or mitral regions.

LABORATORY FINDINGS

Blood: Sedimentation rate increased; leukocytes, 15,000–18,000, with increase in polymorphonuclears (80–90 per cent); possibly, eosinophilia (up to 9 to 12 per cent).

Electrocardiogram: Possibly, evidence of defect in conduction system.

CLINICAL COURSE: Spectacular response to salicylates (polyarticular rheumatism) or chemotherapy (early gonococcic type).

BIBLIOGRAPHY

BERGER, H.: Intermittent Hydrarthrosis with Allergic Basis, J. A. M. A. 112:2402–2405, 1939.

GUTMANN, M. J.: Allergy in Relation to Arthritis, M. Rec. 147:204–208, 1938.

KINSELLA, R. A: Differential Diagnosis of Acute Rheumatic Fever, J. Lab. & Clin. Med. 22:26–29, 1936.

MOURIQUAND, G.: L'allergie dans les maladies rhumatismales [Allergy in rheumatic diseases], Acta rheumatol. 8:8–14, 1936.

PORTER, J. L., AND LONERGAN, R. C.: Intermittent Hydrarthrosis, J. Bone & Joint Surg. 14:631–639, 1932.

POTTENGER, R. T.: Constitutional Factors in Arthritis with Special Reference to Incidence and Rôle of Allergic Diseases, Ann. Int. Med. 12:323–333, 1938.

TROUT, E. F., AND VRTIAK, E. G.: Statistical Study of Allergy in Arthritis, Ann. Int. Med. 13:761–767, 1939.

TZANCK, A.; LAYANI, F.; SIDI, E., AND KLOTZ, H. P.: Les rhumatismes de la chimiothérapie [Rheumatism due to intolerance to chemotherapy], Presse méd. 44:1052–1055, 1936.

WOOTTON, W. T.: Rôle of Allergy in Arthritis, J. Arkansas M. Soc. 32:119–122, 1936.

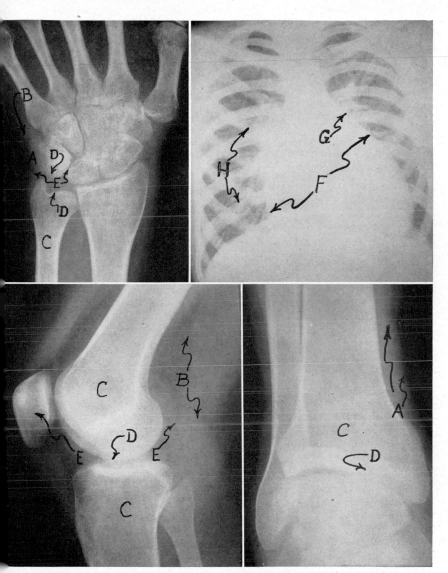

Figs. 262–265.—Multiple joint involvement with no tendency to bilaterality is the rule for all types of allergic arthritis. There may be localized swelling of soft tissues, A; localized edema, B; normal osseous architecture, C; normal osseous articular cortexes, D; possibly, slight expansion of interosseous spacing, E. Particularly with definite toxic manifestations such as fever, leukocytosis and palpable subcutaneous nodules, rheumatic fever is to be suspected. Study of the heart may reveal "rheumatic configuration," with enlargement of the oblique diameter, F; prominence in the region of the conus and base of the pulmonary arteries, G; possibly, evidence of pulmonary congestion, H.

Rheumatoid Arthritis: Juvenile Type

SYNONYMS: Chronic arthritis of childhood, rheumatoid arthritis of childhood, Still's disease, Chauffard-Still's disease.

ROENTGEN CRITERIA

EARLY STAGES

Soft tissues: Fusiform swellings with obliteration of fascial planes.
Regional bones: Slight deossification.
Articular cortexes: Slight deossification.
Joint space: Expanded; possibly, increased spacing between extremities of the osseous articular cortexes.

LATER STAGES

Soft tissues: Atrophy.
Regional bones: Progressive deossification with thinning of trabeculations; possibly, cortical and subarticular cortical cysts; possibly, premature ossification of epiphyses.
Articular cortexes: Likely, flattened; possibly, smooth irregularities.
Joint space: Reduced; possibly, cleavage line (fibrous ankylosis); possibly, osseous bridging; possibly, subluxations.

CORROBORATIVE ROENTGEN CRITERIA: Bilateral symmetrical involvement of knees, wrists, elbows, ankles, fingers, hips; possibly, evidence of pericardial effusion or adhesions; possibly, enlarged spleen or liver.

INCIDENCE

Age: Acute episodes as early as 3-10 years (case reported in infant of 4 months).
Sex: Apparently irrelevant.
Climate: Greatest in temperate zone.

HISTORY: Usually, gradual onset of fever and stiffness of joints, possibly preceded by upper respiratory infection or tonsillitis;

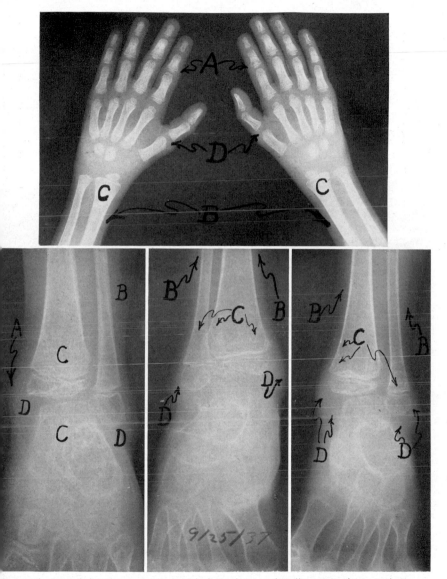

Juvenile rheumatoid arthritis, early stage. Multiple involvement of smaller peripheral joints and characteristic bilaterality. **Figs. 266 (above) and 267 (left below).**—Especially early stage. Periarticular edema, A; soft tissue atrophy, B; delicate osseous architecture, C; widening of joint spaces, D. **Figs. 268 and 269 (center and right below).**—After several months. Conspicuous soft tissue atrophy, B; conspicuous deossification, C; persistent widening of joint space, D.

LABORATORY FINDINGS

Blood: Sedimentation rate increased; white cells early increased, above 10,000, though later reduced to 5,000 or less; differential count variable, polymorphonuclears 14–86 per cent in early stages, with Shilling shift to left; red cell and hemoglobin values below normal (hypochromic anemia).

Basal metabolic rate: Likely, less than −10 (to −60).

Biopsy of subcutaneous nodule: Histologic picture of Aschoff body.

CLINICAL COURSE: Usually, progressive aggravation of joint symptoms and limitation of function over a period of years; possibly, sudden cessation, except for aggravation under conditions of minimal strains or stresses, unless ankylosis has taken place.

BIBLIOGRAPHY

BETHEA, O. W.: Atrophic Arthritis, Internat. M. Digest 36:172–175, 1940.
BOOTS, R. H.: Essential Features in Differential Diagnosis of Rheumatoid and Osteo-Arthritis, J. Lab. & Clin. Med. 22:14–18, 1936.
BREU, W., AND FLEISCHHACKER, H.: Über das Feltysche Syndrom [Felty's Syndrome], Wien. klin. Wchnschr. 51:1081–1087, 1938.
CURTIS, A. C., AND POLLARD, H. M.: Felty's Syndrome: Its Several Features, Including Tissue Changes, Compared with Other Forms of Rheumatoid Arthritis, Ann. Int. Med. 13:2265–2284, 1940.
EDGECOMB, W.: Rheumatoid Arthritis, Brit. M. J. 2:387–391, 1938.
FELTY, A. R.: Chronic Arthritis in Adult Associated with Splenomegaly and Leukopenia, Bull. Johns Hopkins Hosp. 35:16–20, 1924.
FERGUSON, A. S.: Roentgenographic Features of Rheumatoid Arthritis, J. Bone & Joint Surg. 18:297–300, 1936.
FINEMAN, S.: Rôle of the Roentgenologist in Diagnosis and Treatment of Chronic Arthritis, M. Clin. North America 21:1641–1661, 1937.
RIGLER, L., AND WETHERBY, M.: Roentgen Findings in Chronic Polyarticular Arthritis, Am. J. Roentgenol. 29:766–773, 1933.
SPACKMAN, E. W.: Roentgen Aspects of Chronic Arthritis, Am. J. Roentgenol. 35:156–186, 1936.
WAITZKIN, L.: Felty's Syndrome, Virginia M. Monthly 69:80–84, 1942.
WILLIAMS, R. H.: Felty's Syndrome: Report of Case with Necropsy Findings, Ann. Int. Med. 9:1247–1255, 1936.
ZULICK, J. D.: Roentgenographic Aspects of Rheumatoid Diseases, Pennsylvania M. J. 44:1284-1285, 1941.

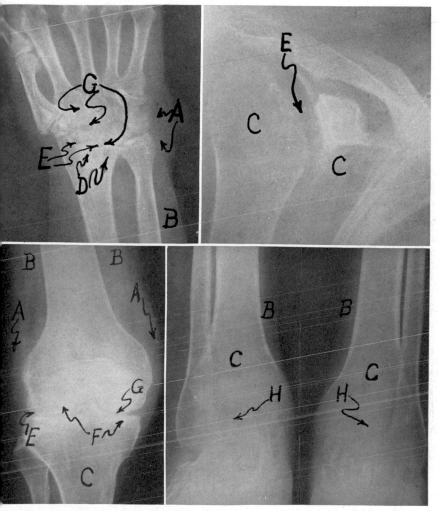

Figs. 286–289.—Moderately advanced stage, emphasizing inflammatory stage. Multiple and bilateral joint involvement prominent. Periarticular edema, *A,* with obliteration of fascial planes; moderate atrophy of muscles, *B;* deossification, *C,* with subarticular cortical cystic changes, *D;* flattening and smooth irregularity of osseous articular cortexes, *E;* slight eburnation, *F,* from weight-bearing and use; reduction of interosseous spacing, i.e., destruction of articular cartilage, *G;* evidence of fibrous ankylosis, i.e., cleavage line, *H.*

Skin test: Tuberculin-positive (of value in young children).
Joint aspiration: Positive guinea-pig inoculation (approximately 80 per cent trustworthy).
Biopsy: Tubercles in synovia or outer sheath of capsule.

CLINICAL COURSE: Alleviation with complete bed rest or with cast fixation for six weeks; reaggravation of symptoms with reactivation or removal of cast (Thomas' test).

BIBLIOGRAPHY

DICKSON, F. D.: Differential Diagnosis of Tuberculosis Arthritis, J. Lab. & Clin. Med. 22:35–43, 1936.
ELLIOTT, A. E.: Tuberculous Cysts of the Knee Joint, Am. J. Roentgenol. 34:209–213, 1935.
FERGUSON, A. B.: Roentgenography of Tuberculosis of Joints, J. Bone & Joint Surg. 19:653–656, 1937.
GIRDLESTONE, G. R.: Pathology and Treatment of Tuberculosis of Knee-Joint, Brit. J. Surg. 19:488–507, 1932.
HENDERSON, M. S.: Tuberculosis of Joints, with Special Reference to Knee, Australian & New Zealand J. Surg. 6:27–36, 1936.
KLEINBERG, S.: Tuberculous Arthritis, M. Clin. North America 21:1723–1737, 1937.
LE COCQ, J. F.: Diagnosis and Treatment of Bone and Joint Tuberculosis, Northwest Med. 38:349–352, 1939.
MCKEEVER, F. M.: Tuberculosis of the Knee in Infancy and Childhood, J. A. M. A. 113:1293–1299, 1939.
PHEMISTER, D. B.: Changes in Articular Surfaces in Tuberculous and in Pyogenic Infections of Joints, Am. J. Roentgenol. 12:1–14, 1924.
———, AND HATCHER, C. H.: Correlation of Pathological and Roentgenological Findings in Diagnosis of Tuberculous Arthritis, Am. J. Roentgenol. 29:736–752, 1933.
POMERANZ, M. M.: Roentgen Diagnosis of Bone and Joint Tuberculosis, Am. J. Roentgenol. 29:753–762, 1933.
NATHANSON, L., AND COHEN, W.: Statistical and Roentgenological Analysis of Two Hundred Cases of Bone and Joint Tuberculosis, Radiology 36:550–567, 1941.
SMITH, A. DE F.: Early Diagnosis of Joint Tuberculosis, J. A. M. A. 83:1569–1573, 1924.

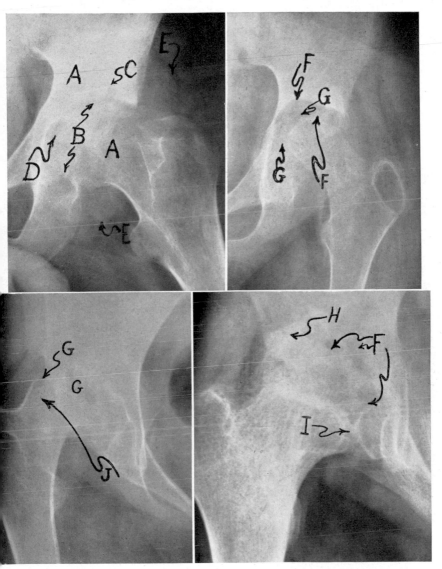

Changes after months of involvement. **Fig. 312 (left above).**—Moderate deossification of regional bones, A; slight deossification of osseous articular cortexes (evidence of *low grade* inflammation, considering the history of prolonged disturbance), B; sequestration, C; conspicuous reduction of interosseous spacing, i.e., destruction of articular cartilages, D, yet widening of true joint space, E. **Fig. 313 (right above).**—Dissolution of osseous articular cortexes, F; actual osteomyelitic process, G. **Figure 314 (left below)** shows a luxation, J, while **Figure 315 (right below)** shows a "burned-out" process with evidence of ankylosis, both fibrous, i.e., cleavage line, H, and osseous, I.

INCIDENCE

Age: Approximately 60 per cent between 20 and 30; 30 per cent between 30 and 40; otherwise, prior to 20 and after 40.

Sex: Approximately two-thirds in males.

Joints involved: Usually weight-bearing, such as knee or ankle. Accounts for approximately 2 per cent of "rheumatics"; joint symptoms occur in about 1 per cent of all gonorrheal infections.

HISTORY: Background of gonorrhea; possibly, complications and symptomatology of prostatitis or salpingitis; thereafter or concurrently, preliminary involvement of joints by "fleeting polyarthritis" with transient stiffness, swelling and slight pain on movement; ultimately, localization with extreme swelling, agonizing pain and tenderness in one or a few joints, likely ushered in with malaise, chills and generalized aching.

PHYSICAL FINDINGS: Likely, good physical condition (relatively acute onset); swelling with redness and increased temperature around one or a few joints, with limitation of voluntary movement and guarding against passive movement because of extreme pain, usually, and tenderness on digital pressure; temperature likely 99–101 F.; possibly, tender and enlarged lymph nodes.

LABORATORY FINDINGS

Blood: Leukocytes 50,000–60,000; differential count high in polymorphonuclears, 85–90 per cent; serum proteins elevated, 6 or more Gm. per 100 cc.; sedimentation rate increased.

Complement fixation test: Positive in 40 per cent six weeks and up to two years after onset.

Urethral smears: Likely, positive for gram-negative intracellular diplococci.

Joint aspirations: Smears positive in 30 per cent; possibly, positive culture (best results during first six days of acute symptoms). Complement fixation test may be positive (in approximately 85 per cent six weeks to six months or longer following onset).

Joint biopsy: Gonococci in synovia.

Skin test: Positive in approximately 90 per cent.

Electrocardiogram: Likely, increased P-R interval (to 0.21 second).

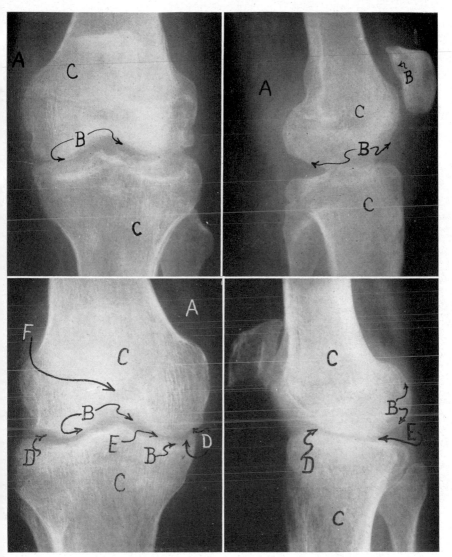

Figs. 335–338.—The intense inflammatory and destructive characteristics of gonococcic arthritis are evident in marked periarticular edema, A; conspicuous deossification of osseous articular cortexes, B, in contrast to more normal architecture at a distance from the joint, C (signifying usage until recent disturbance); early erosion of osseous articular cortexes, D, with reduction of interosseous spacing, E (signifying destruction of articular cartilage), and possibly subluxation, F.

Infectious Arthritis: Syphilitic

SYNONYMS: Chondro-osteo-arthritis, Förster's arthritis, Fournier's arthritis, von Gies's polyarthritis, in congenital and heredotypes with infantile tabes—symmetrical hydrarthrosis, Clutton's joints.

ROENTGEN CRITERIA

EARLY STAGES

Soft tissues: Localized swelling, periarticular and perhaps regional to osseous prominences; low grade edema with partial obliteration of fascial planes.

Regional bones: Periosteal proliferations, "whiskered" or scalloped in type, likely to obliterate trabeculation pattern; possibly, endosteal proliferations with reduction in medullary spacing.

Articular cortexes: Likely, dense but hazy (due to early thickening of synovial membrane and perichondrium and to synovial effusion).

Joint space: Expanded, with distention of capsule and deviation of regional tissues, and, possibly, increased interosseous spacing.

LATER STAGES

Soft tissues: Residual periarticular swelling and edema; possibly, slight atrophy.

Regional bones: Periosteal proliferations, especially at osseous extremities; possibly, periosteal "whiskering" or tuftings at sites of ligamentous attachments; possibly, superficial or even more deeply located erosions or destruction, although bone production with appearance of sclerosis is usually predominant.

Articular cortexes: Deossification; possibly, actual erosions; perhaps, sequestrations.

Joint space: Likely, widened with increased interosseous spacing; rarely, narrowed with production of cleavage line or calcifications in synovia; occasionally, calcifications in articular cartilages.

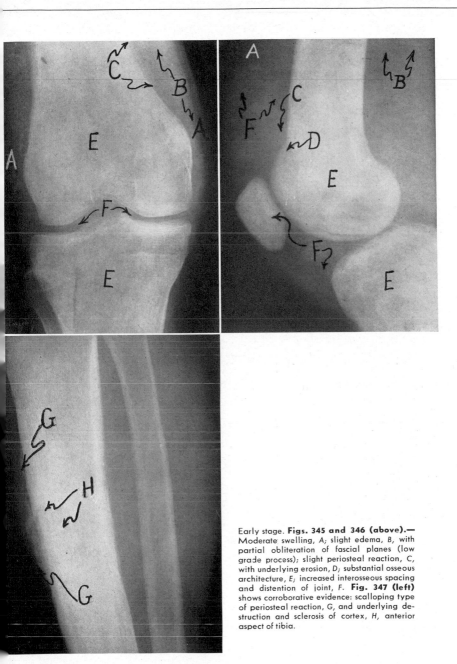

Early stage. **Figs. 345 and 346 (above).—**
Moderate swelling, A; slight edema, B, with
partial obliteration of fascial planes (low
grade process); slight periosteal reaction, C,
with underlying erosion, D; substantial osseous
architecture, E; increased interosseous spacing
and distention of joint, F. **Fig. 347 (left)**
shows corroborative evidence: scalloping type
of periosteal reaction, G, and underlying destruction and sclerosis of cortex, H, anterior
aspect of tibia.

Joint aspirations: Fluid usually clear, with high count of lymphocytes and monocytes and positive complement fixation.

Biopsy of synovial membrane: Conspicuous thickening, with endothelial proliferations and perivascular infiltration of lymphocytes.

CLINICAL COURSE: Spectacular response to antisyphilitic therapy; subsidence of fever 24–48 hours thereafter; progressive reduction of joint manifestations; roentgen evidence of healing in one month, with restoration of normal architecture in 4 to 6 months; possibly, residual calcifications in synovial membrane or articular cartilages with or without eburnations and spurs.

BIBLIOGRAPHY

CAMPBELL, W. C.: Analysis of Bone and Joint Lesions of Known Syphilitic Origin, Radiology 5:122–131, 1925.

COMPERE, E. L.: Syphilis of Bones and Joints, Urol. & Cutan. Rev. 44:535–540, 1940.

COMROE, B. I.: Syphilitic Joint Disease, Urol. & Cutan. Rev. 46:234–236, 1942.

KLAUDER, J. V., AND ROBERTSON, H. F.: Symmetrical Serous Synovitis (Clutton's Joints): Congenital Syphilis and Keratitis, J. A. M. A. 103:236–240, 1934.

KLING, D. H.: Syphilitic Arthritis with Effusion, Am. J. M. Sc. 183:538–549, 1932.

LAMB, H. W.: Bone and Joint Syphilis, J. Maine M. A. 20:47–52, 1929.

McEWEN, C., AND THOMAS, E. W.: Syphilitic Joint Disease, M. Clin. North America 22:1275–1286, 1938.

SPEED, J. S., AND BOYD, H. B.: Bone Syphilis, South. M. J. 29:371–377, 1936.

WILE, U. J., AND SENEAR, F. E.: Study of Involvement of Bones and Joints in Early Syphilis, Am. J. M. Sc. 152:689–693, 1916.

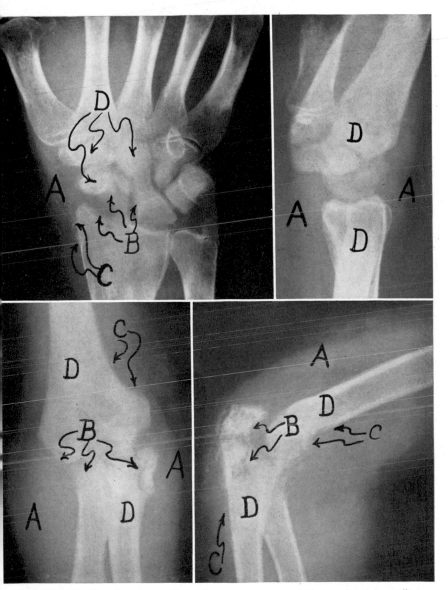

Figs. 352–355.—Very late stage—still an inflammatory process, as evident in *periarticular* swelling *and* edema of soft tissues, A, and destruction of osseous articular cortexes, B. Deossification such as usually associated with inflammation is lacking; instead, note periosteal "whiskering," C, and sclerosis of bones, D.

Gout

SYNONYMS: Gouty arthritis, arthritis urica, uratic arthritis, tophaceous arthritis, podagra, metabolic arthritis, goutte, gicht, gota, painful big toe.

ROENTGEN CRITERIA

EARLY STAGES

Likely to mimic allergic arthritis; later, early rheumatoid arthritis.

Soft tissues: Edema, with peri- or para-arthritic obliterations of fascial planes.

Regional bones: Likely, normal.

Articular cortexes: Likely, normal; possibly, beginning cortical cystic dissolutions; possibly, beginning eburnations.

Joint space: Likely, expanded.

LATER STAGES

Soft tissues: During acute episodes: likely, localized edema with para-arthritic obliterations of fascial planes; possibly, edematous outline of tendons or bursae (i.e., olecranon or metatarsal). Possibly, localized tumefactions, with or without calcifications; likely, lineal streak of calcifications in arteries or disklike densities due to phleboliths.

Regional bones: Likely, coarsened trabeculation pattern; possibly, cystic dissolutions between trabeculation architecture; possibly, periosteal tuftings.

Articular cortexes: Eburnations; cortical and subcortical cystic dissolutions; marginal spurs, possibly to the extent of "basket-weave overlay"; possibly, fragmentations of these spurs; irregularities in osseous articular surfaces.

Joint space: Likely, widened at periphery (during acute episodes); reduction in interosseous spacing (because of destruction of articular cartilages); possibly, subluxations.

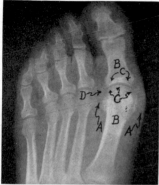

Figs. 380–382.—Relatively early stage. After years of intermittent episodes of acute joint swellings and pain, roentgen study may show: localized peri- or para-articular swelling, especially around first metatarsal joint, *A;* architecture of regional bones normal or coarsened, *B;* slight cortical cystic dissolutions, *C;* widening of joint space, *D* (later, reduction and decrease of interosseous spacing, *E*).

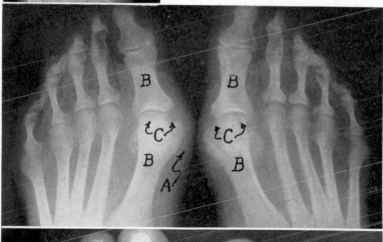

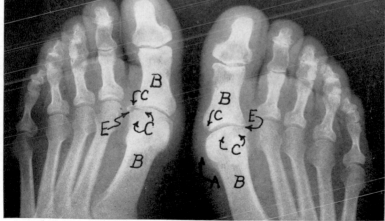

CORROBORATIVE ROENTGEN CRITERIA: Early manifestations usually apparent in several joints, but no tendency toward bilateral symmetry. Later, metatarso- or interphalangeal joints of big toe involved in 60 to 75 per cent; otherwise, metacarpo- or interphalangeal joints of hands or knees, ankles or elbows are most frequently involved.

INCIDENCE

Age: Earliest manifestations usually during thirties; possibly, even twenties or earlier; typical roentgen manifestations rare prior to 40.

Sex: Males predominantly involved (90–98 per cent).

Heredity: Sufficiently related that one should inquire as to "intermittent arthritis" in father of any suspect subject.

Race: Almost exclusively among whites, especially English and Americans (rare among yellow race).

Type of individual: Robust, athletic, heavy eater and steady drinker.

Occupation: Frequently, contact with lead.

Frequency: Constitutes 5–8 per cent of cases in American arthritic clinics.

HISTORY: First attacks are seldom correctly diagnosed. Likely, 10–15 years of intermittent attacks of fever, joint pains, swellings and intense inflammation, having abrupt onset and almost as abrupt termination, these episodes likely to have involved many joints; prolonged sinus drainage not very uncommon. Bilaterality and symmetry the rule; acute symptoms characteristically last 3–10 days. Such attacks occur particularly during spring or fall and may be precipitated by mental or physical fatigue, trauma or a gastrointestinal disturbance; occasionally, precipitated by therapy for some coincident disease (cases reported in connection with liver therapy for anemia; ketogenic diet for bacilluria; use of salyrgan, gynergen, insulin, etc.) There may be background of renal colic (10–15 per cent have urate deposits). Later, attacks occur at shorter and shorter intervals and episodes of joint distress are usually described as more and more prolonged. After 12 to 15 years, achings are likely to become more chronic, with localization to a few joints— metatarsophalangeals of the big toes, metacarpophalangeals, interphalangeals, wrists or elbows.

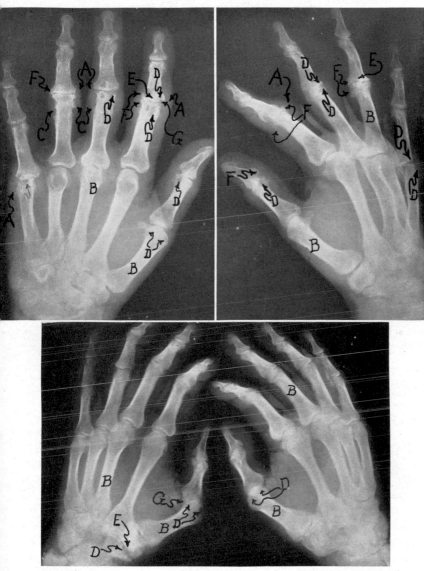

Figs. 383–385.—Moderately advanced stage, with changes in hands and wrists. Periarticular swelling and edema, *A;* substantial architecture of bones, *B;* periosteal tufts, *C;* cortical and subcortical cystic dissolution, *D;* eburnation, *E;* marginal spur formation, *F;* reduction of interosseous spacing, G. Note multiplicity of involvement. Bilaterality is the rule.

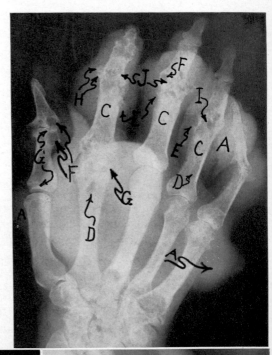

Figs. 392–394.—Late stage. Soft tissue tumefactions, *A,* featuring tophi; streaks of calcific densities, *B,* indicating sclerosis of vessels; coarsened trabeculation pattern of bones, *C,* with cystic deossifications, *D,* consistent with limitation of use; periosteal tufting, *E;* cortical and subcortical cystic dissolutions, *F,* representing subcartilaginous deposits of urates; eburnations, *G;* marginal spurs, *H;* marked irregularity of osseous articular cortexes, *I;* obliteration of interosseous spacing, *J,* signifying destruction of articular cartilages.

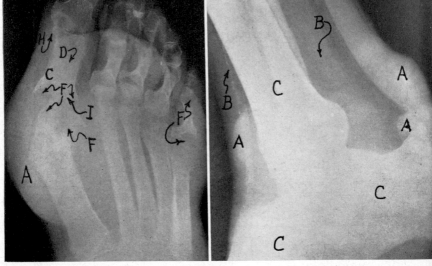

Neoplasms: Peripheral Joints

FEW STRUCTURES within the confines of joints and their lining membranes are susceptible to neoplastic change. Tissues which may be involved include the synovial membrane, its vascular bed and fat deposits. Apparently, the articular cartilages are exempt from primary neoplastic changes (except for the rare occurrence of "myxomatous cysts" in the menisci of the knee).

Following the usual classification of neoplastic lesions, when found in the bones themselves, one might classify neoplasms of joints as either benign or malignant. However, in the case of the joints, each group appears to be represented at least roentgenologically by a single entity: the benign, by osteochondromatosis; the malignant, by synoviomas.

Particularly when there is bulging of the joint capsule, with no evidence of periarticular edema, the possibility of neoplasm must be considered. This diagnosis should be especially prominent in one's mind if clinically there is a history of gradual but progressive limitation of function of that joint, possibly intermittent locking and notable absence of local inflammation or general toxic state.

One can hardly be enthusiastic about the roentgenographic evidence of these lesions during the earliest stages. The tissues, regardless of type of joint neoplasm, are ray transparent. Even in the case of osteochondromatosis, which is easily demonstrable later, the initial changes are merely of hypertrophy of synovial membrane—a ray-transparent medium. Even after villous formations appear it may be impossible to distinguish this condition from fatty deposits, actual lipomas, hemangiomas, xanthomas (giant cell tumors of the synovia), or even the small myxomatous cyst of an intra-articular disk (all of which are possibilities as benign tumors). Later, of course, osteochondromatosis is distinguished by metaplasia of the synovial villous tissue into cartilage and thereafter by calcifications and ossifications, which are easily visualized roentgenographically. Then, of course, the findings are distinctive.

Malignant changes of the five types of benign tumors mentioned above are not known to me. This statement is presented tentatively as a challenge to identify such. Otherwise, the synovioma appears to be the only type of malignant tumor arising *within* a joint. Perhaps it represents malignant change after synovial hypertrophy —a malignant variant of what otherwise would become osteochondromatosis.

Both benign and malignant tumors arising from the bones proper may invade the joints or at least embarrass their mechanical function. To provide a warning that joint symptoms might be due to such, various examples of bone tumors of this character are presented, though detailed descriptions are not included since they are more pertinent to a dissertation on bones per se.

Osteochondromatosis

SYNONYMS: Synovial osteochondromatosis, enchondromas of the joint cavity, chondromatosis, chondromas of synovial membrane.

ROENTGEN CRITERIA

EARLY STAGES
  Soft tissues: Likely, normal.
  Regional bones: Possibly, evidence of old fracture.
  Articular cortexes: Likely, normal.
  Joint space: Possibly, merely widened with bulging of capsule. (The intra-articular bodies may be composed entirely of synovium or of fibrous tissue and cartilage with no evidence of calcific deposits, therefore ray transparent.) Possibly, calcific inclusions, usually disklike, with calcific concentrations at periphery and in center of each.

LATER STAGES
  Soft tissues: Likely, normal.
  Regional bones: Possibly, evidence of old fracture.
  Articular cortexes: Possibly, eburnation, marginal spur formations and irregularities in osseous articular cortexes.

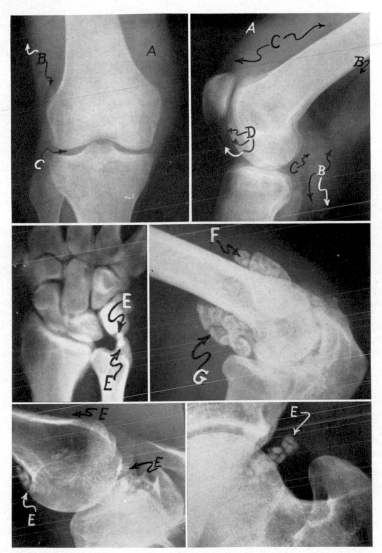

Intra-articular neoplasms are featured by tumefaction, *A*; distinct fascial planes, *B* (contradicting infection); expansion of joint space, indicated by bulging of capsule, increased interosseous spacing and anterosuperior displacement of patella, *C*. **Figures 395 and 396 (top)** show these changes, consistent not only with early stages of osteochondromatosis (proved by exploration in this case) but with lipomas, xanthomas, synoviomas and even cartilage cysts. Note slight flecking of calcification, *D*. This may be found with osteochondromatosis, hemangioma and synovioma. **Figures 397–400 (center and bottom)** show well developed osteochondromatosis in various joints. Typical rice bodies, *E*, with calcific condensations in their centers, *F*, and around the peripheries, *G*.

Joint space: Likely, expanded, with definite bulging of capsule; inclusion of calcific densities of disklike configuration having greatest densities at periphery and in center of each.

CORROBORATIVE ROENTGEN CRITERIA: Changes may be found in any joint (usually monarticular), but most common in knee, elbow, hip, shoulder and wrist. Likely, associated evidence of trauma—old fracture or osteo-arthropathy or results of hemorrhage.

INCIDENCE
Age: Most patients between 25 and 50.
Sex: Approximately 75 per cent in males.
Occupation: Usually arduous or hazardous as to falls (trauma reported in approximately 50 per cent).

HISTORY: Frequently, trauma; later, notice of limitation in range of movement of the particular joint; possibly, locking of joint; occasionally, sharp aching.

PHYSICAL FINDINGS: Patient usually healthy appearing, with no evidence of fever or toxicity; possibly, obvious limitation of use of involved joints but, likely, no definite guarding of it. The joint may be prominent but without redness or pitting edema. On palpation, capsule likely to feel boggy and minute bodies may be palpable, even to the extent of their gliding around in it. Tenderness is not the rule, even on deep palpation.

LABORATORY FINDINGS: Irrelevant except for:
Biopsy of synovia: Likely, marked thickening, with villous proliferation in which there may be cartilage and, possibly, calcium or actual bone. Lymphocytic infiltration may be scattered throughout.

CLINICAL COURSE: Progressive limitation of joint function with intermittent locking; improvement following removal of cartilaginous bodies, with possible recurrence until adequate synovectomy.

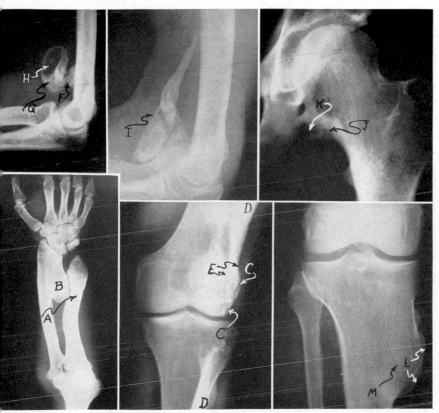

Extra-articular anomalies and neoplasms may limit joint function owing to mechanical factors. **Fig. 401 (left above).**—Subperiosteal hemorrhage. Pedicle attachment to bone, *F;* peripheral lamination of calcification, *G;* central area of incomplete organization, *H.* **Fig. 402 (center above).**—Myositis ossificans. Calcified sheath extending into and between muscle bundles, *I.* **Fig. 403 (right above).**—Osteochondroma. Continuity of cortex through base, *J;* ray-transparent cartilaginous cap, *K.* **Fig. 404 (left below).**—Derangement of wrist due to chondrodysplasia. Deviation of ulna, *A,* because of exostosis, *B.* **Fig. 405 (center below).**—Melorheostosis Leri. Superficial cortical erosions, *C,* simulating erosion by infection; flowing type of hyperostosis, *D;* widening of cortex, *E.* **Fig. 406 (right below).**—Osteoma. Intact cortex, *L;* continuity of trabeculations, *M.* Such conditions are likely to cause maldevelopment of muscle bundles; therefore, malsupport by opposing groups, malalinement of bones, abnormal joint function and secondary osteo-arthropathic changes.

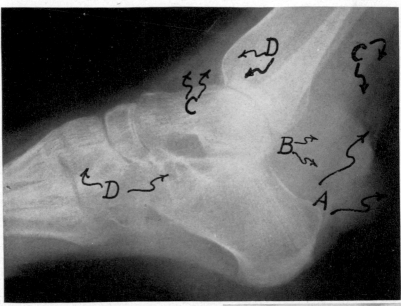

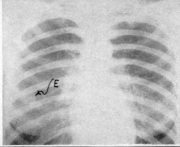

Fig. 416 (top).—Synovioma of ankle. Nodular tumefaction, A; slight calcific speckling, B; distinct fascial planes (contradicting infection), C; slight deossification of regional bones (limited use), D. **Fig. 417 (middle).**—At this stage, metastasis, E, was noted in the lung. **Fig. 418 (below).**—Synovioma in knee (commonest site), with similar findings, tumefaction, A, distinct fascial planes, B.

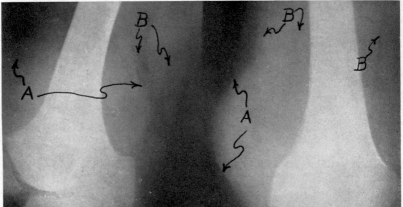

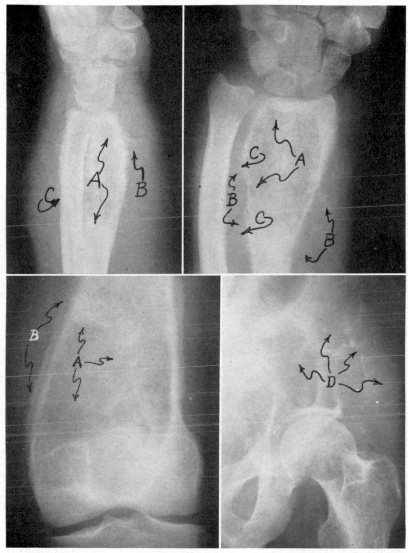

Malignant lesions in bone are likely to produce pains interpreted as due to joint pathology. **Figs. 419 and 420 (above) and 421 (left below).**—Malignant giant cell tumors. Note soft tissue tumefaction, as in synovioma, but with epiphyseal involvement, as with the benign type of giant cell tumor but, in contrast to the latter, note paucity of basket-weave scaffolding, *A*, and periosteal reaction, *B*. In **Figures 419 and 420,** there is evidence of a break through the cortex, *C*. Similar destruction of osseous articular cortex may occur, with invasion of joint space. **Fig. 422 (right below).**—Similar lesion but a truly vascular tumor, endothelioma. Note multilocularity of osseous residuum, *D*. This lesion eventually extended into the joint, with collapse of osseous articular cortex.

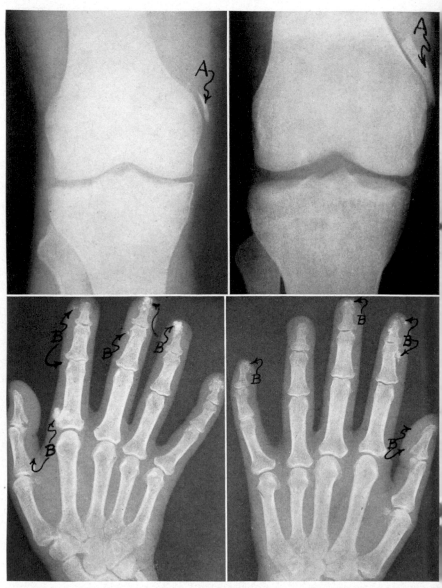

Calcific deposits may be found around joints, such as the knee, after trauma. **Figs. 439 and 440 (above).** —"Pellegrini-Stieda's disease," with calcification, A, around the internal condylar ligament or tendons of the adductor magnus or vastus medialis. More superficially located calcifications, B in **Figures 441 and 442 (below),** may be found in cases of dermoliths, chalk gout and scleroderma and occasionally in Addison's disease. These may reduce function of regional joints.

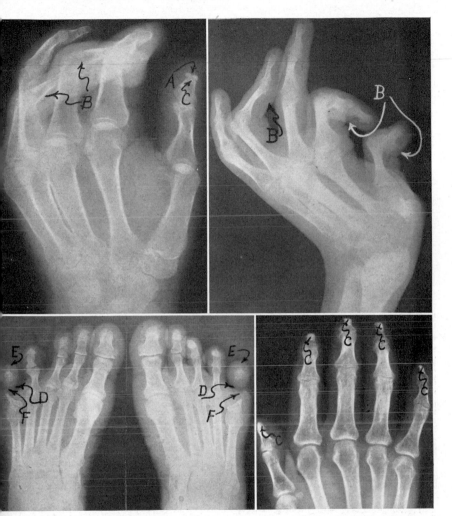

In scleroderma **(Fig. 443, left above),** in addition to subcutaneous calcifications, A, and occasionally intramuscular calcifications, there are also contractures, B, and absorption of ungual tufts, C. Contractures may be due to stenosis of a tendon sheath (in which case only one or a few tendons are involved), to Dupuytren's involvement or to muscle atrophy, as produced by poliomyelitis **(Fig. 444, right above).** In ainhum **(Fig. 445, left below),** absorption of ungual tufts may occur in the fifth digits of the feet; there are annular constriction, D, and absorption not only of the ungual tufts, E, but of other portions of bone, F, even to the degree found in leprosy (auto-amputation may occur). Absorption of ungual tufts may occur in Raynaud's disease **(Fig. 446, right below).**

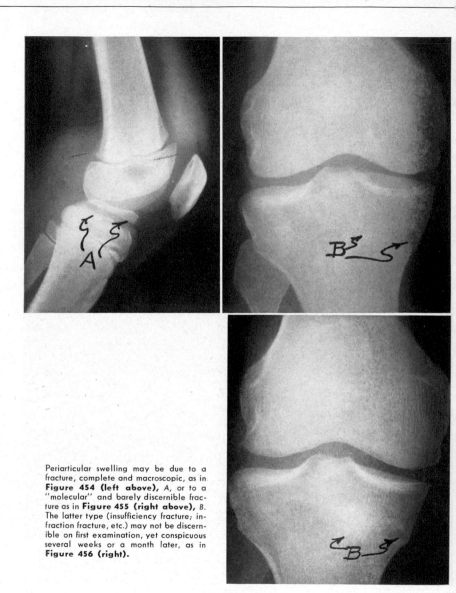

Periarticular swelling may be due to a fracture, complete and macroscopic, as in **Figure 454 (left above)**, *A*, or to a "molecular" and barely discernible fracture as in **Figure 455 (right above)**, *B*. The latter type (insufficiency fracture; infraction fracture, etc.) may not be discernible on first examination, yet conspicuous several weeks or a month later, as in **Figure 456 (right)**.

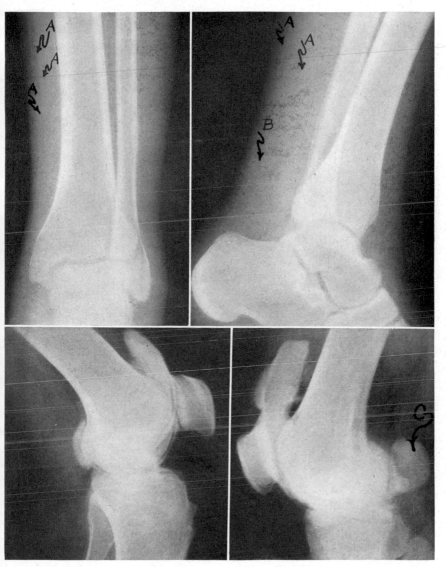

Swellings around small joints of hands or feet or even around larger joints of the extremities, such as the ankle, may be due to cardiac or kidney pathology **(Figs. 457 and 458, above).** Note obliteration of fascial planes, A, and complete obliteration of the posterior triangle, B, as found with inflammation; but there is no evidence of deossification generally or regional to the joints. Localized swelling may be due to herniation of the synovial membrane, as in Baker's cyst. **Fig. 459 (left below).**—Filling of a normal knee joint with radiopaque medium (diodrast). **Fig. 460 (right below).**—The outpocketing, C— Baker's cyst.

BIBLIOGRAPHY

BERCOW, C., AND POPPEL, M. H.: Interstitial Calcinosis Circumscripta Associated with Scleroderma and Raynaud's Disease, Radiology 39:96–98, 1942.

CAFFEY, J.: Skeletal Changes after Administration of Bismuth, Am. J. Roentgenol. 37:405–406, 1937.

COLEY, B. L., AND MOORE, M., JR.: Caisson Disease with Special Reference to Bones and Joints: 2 Cases, Ann. Surg. 111:1065–1075, 1940.

COOPER, W.: Calcareous Tendinitis in Metacarpophalangeal Region, J. Bone & Joint Surg. 24:114–122, 1942.

CUSHING, E. H.: "Club Fingers" and Hypertrophic Pulmonary Osteoarthropathy, Internat. Clin. 2:200–205, 1937.

DE LORIMIER, A. A.: Roentgen Therapy in Acute Para-Arthritis, Am. J. Roentgenol. 38:178–195, 1937.

DOWLING, G. B., AND GRIFFITHS, W. J.: Dermatomyositis and Progressive Scleroderma, Lancet 1:1424–1428, 1939.

FREUND, E.: Idiopathic Familial Generalized Osteophytosis, Am. J. Roentgenol. 39:216–227, 1938.

KAHLSTROM, S. C.: Bone Infarcts, Am. J. Roentgenol. 47:405–416, 1942.

KEY, J. A.: Foreign Body Arthritis, Surg., Gynec. & Obst. 70:897–902, 1940.

LERICHE, R.: Problem of Osteo-Articular Diseases of Vasomotor Origin: Hydrarthrosis and Traumatic Arthritis: Genesis and Treatment, J. Bone & Joint Surg. 10:492–500, 1928.

LONGCOPE, W. T., AND PIERSON, J. W.: Boeck's Sarcoid (Sarcoidosis), Bull. Johns Hopkins Hosp. 60:223–298, 1937.

ODESSKY, J. W., AND SHIRSHNER, P. A.: Generalized Ossifying Periostitis: Report of Case, Radiology 30:250–254, 1938.

PODKAMINSKIY, N. A.: Acrosclerosis Hyperplastica Intra-Ossea, Am. J. Roentgenol. 38:889–892, 1937.

SANDSTRÖM, C.: Peritendinitis Calcarea: Common Disease of Middle Life: Its Diagnosis, Pathology and Treatment, Am. J. Roentgenol. 40:1–21, 1938.

SHAPIRO, S.: Ossifying Periostitis of Bamberger-Marie (Secondary Hypertrophic Pulmonary Osteoarthropathy), Bull. Hosp. Joint Dis. 2:77–83, 1941.

SLOCUMB, C. H.: Differential Diagnosis of Periarticular Fibrositis and Arthritis, J. Lab. & Clin. Med. 22:56–63, 1936.

VOGT, E. C.: Roentgenological Diagnosis of Lead Poisoning in Infants and Children, J. A. M. A. 98:125–129, 1932.

PART II

The Joints of the Spine

Normal Developments, Malformations and Pathologic Changes in the Spinal Column

IN THE human embryo, the earliest evidence of an axial column is the formation of a longitudinal groove with its parasagittal ridges of ectodermal tissue—the neural groove and the neural folds. The ventral aspect of the neural groove extends to close proximity with entodermal tissues. The latter then develop a rodlike fold in parallel relationship. This fold becomes the notochord.

Almost as soon as this entodermal rod is formed, mesenchymal tissues grow around it, separating it both from the overlying ectodermal tissues and from the entodermal tissues of the alimentary tract below. Thus the notochord becomes a distinct structure. It serves as a preliminary axial support in the development of vertebrates and as the sole spinal splint for lower forms. It extends from the level of the future midbrain, in the region where the sella turcica later develops, to a level consistent with the extremity of the future coccyx. Abnormalities in the development of the notochord may occur anywhere throughout its length, although malignant changes in notochordal rests (chordomas) usually arise at either of its extremities—the sacrococcygeal region or the skull; in the latter, they occur particularly near the clivus and possibly in the occipital fossa.

This development of the notochord occurs about the second week of fetal life. The ectodermal ridges fuse along their dorsal crests soon thereafter, and together they produce the brain and spinal cord. The mesenchymal tissues described as enveloping the notochord likewise envelop these ectodermal folds and separate them not only from the notochord but also from the more dorsally located ectodermal tissues. The latter eventually develop into skin.

About the end of the second week, the enveloping mesenchymal

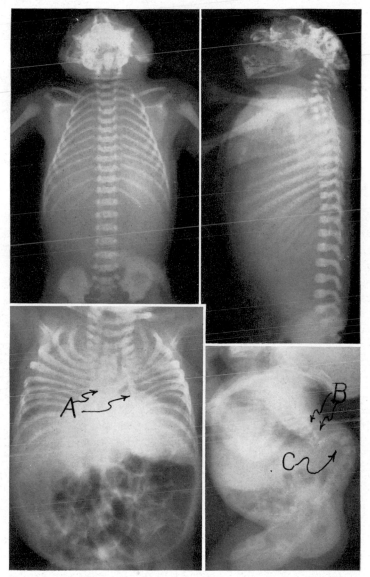

Figs. 468 and 469 (above).—Anencephaly, a defect occurring in the earliest stage of embryonic development—formation of neural groove. **Figs. 470 and 471 (below).**—Myelocele, a defect occurring at a slightly later stage—development of the notochord and, thereafter, mesenchymal envelopment of the notochord and neural ectoderm. Note failure of union of mesenchymal derivative of centra, A; lack of development of laminae, B; conspicuous thoracolumbar hump, C, concerned with the vertebrae. This type of defect is often associated with anencephaly or hydrocephalus and may be diagnosed ante partum.

one for each side; one for the extremity of the spinous process; two for the centrum—one for its upper and one for its lower surface; and, possibly, four for the articular processes—one for each tip. These may not fuse with the central osseous masses until as late as the twenty-fifth year. Particularly prior to that time, and in some individuals even later, these centers may be mistaken for fractures, especially those concerned with the articular processes of the lower thoracic or upper lumbar regions, where the composite densities in the roentgenogram may be confusing. Those concerned with the transverse processes of lumbar vertebrae may be misinterpreted as calculi in the kidneys or urinary tract. They should be distinguished rather easily, though, by their rounded and smooth borders, similar to those of the adjacent extremity of the main portion of the bone.

A similar deficiency of ossification is not uncommonly found in the interarticular zone (the isthmus) of the lower lumbar spine and sacrum. It appears to be the basis for anterior slipping of the upper portion of the spine and the development of a spondylolisthesis.

Thus the development of the spine is highly complicated. These many steps incur numerous possibilities of abnormality. Of all portions of the skeleton, probably none is more subject to nature's mistakes than the spine. *Many* cases of joint deficiency in the spine warrant first consideration of developmental malformations.

BIBLIOGRAPHY

BAILEY, W.: Persistent Vertebral Process Epiphyses, Am. J. Roentgenol. 42:85–90, 1939.

CHAMBERLAIN, W. E.: Basilar Impression (Platybasia), Yale J. Biol. & Med. 11:487–496, 1939.

EHRENHAFT, J. L.: Development of Vertebral Column As Related to Certain Congenital and Pathological Changes, Surg., Gynec. & Obst. 76:282–292, 1943.

FERGUSON, A. B.: Clinical and Roentgenographic Interpretation of Lumbosacral Anomalies, Radiology 22:548–558, 1934.

HUBENY, M., AND DELANO, P. J.: Dysostosis Multiplex, Am. J. Roentgenol. 46:336–342, 1941.

KRAUSE, G. R.: Persistence of Notochord, Am. J. Roentgenol. 44:719–725, 1940.

MEYERDING, H. W.: Diagnosis and Roentgenologic Evidence in Spondylolisthesis, Radiology 20:108–120, 1933.

RUGGLES, H. E.: Dwarfism Due to Disordered Epiphyseal Development, Am. J. Roentgenol. 25:91–94, 1931.

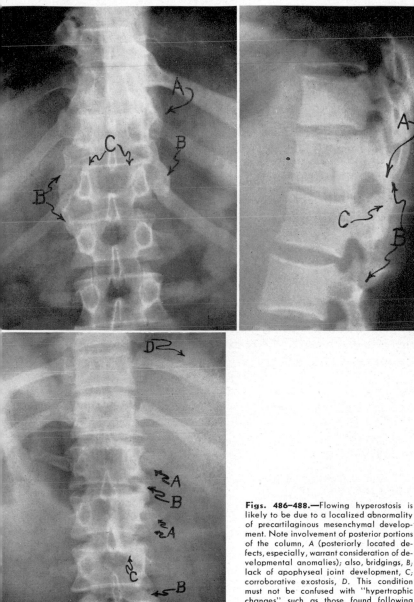

Figs. 486–488.—Flowing hyperostosis is likely to be due to a localized abnormality of precartilaginous mesenchymal development. Note involvement of posterior portions of the column, A (posteriorly located defects, especially, warrant consideration of developmental anomalies); also, bridgings, B; lack of apophyseal joint development, C; corroborative exostosis, D. This condition must not be confused with "hypertrophic changes" such as those found following trauma or abnormal stress.

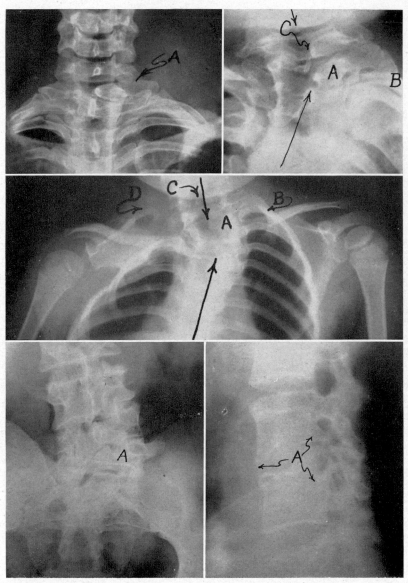

Figs. 489–493.—Scoliosis produced by supernumerary derivatives for centra, A, one type of wedge-shaped vertebrae. Note posterior location of abnormalities. In thoracic region, note associated supernumerary ribs, B, and corroborative findings of failure of fusion of laminae, C, and Sprengel's deformity, D, emphasizing tendency to multiplicity of defects when any one occurs.

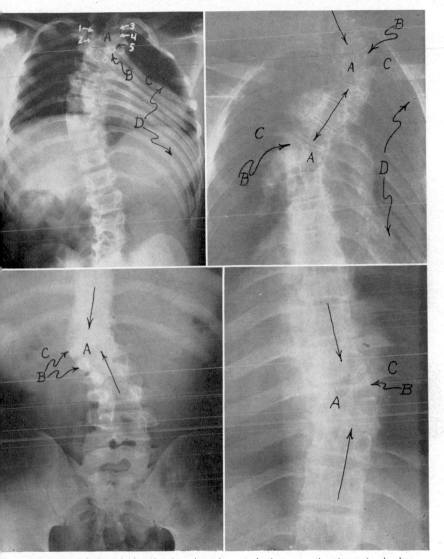

Figs. 494–497.—Scoliosis from wedge-shaped vertebrae, A. In these cases, there is oversize development because of fusion of five instead of the usual four mesenchymal precursors. Supernumerary portions, B; associated supernumerary ribs or transverse processes, C; deformity of thoracic cage, D. In **Figure 494 (left above),** there has been fusion of five precursors—equivalent to two vertebrae plus a supernumerary segment. In **Figure 495 (right above),** note abnormality at two levels.

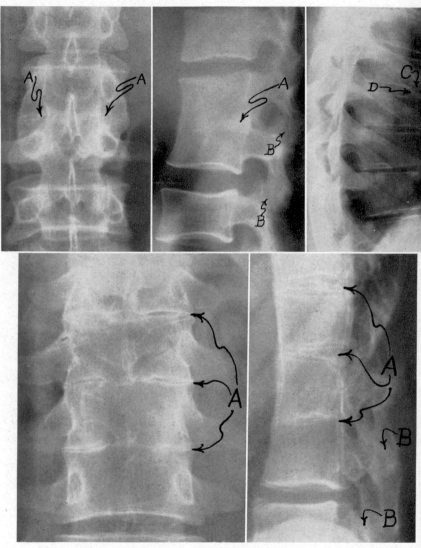

Figs. 498–502.—"Block vertebrae," the result of failure of joint formation between centra—failure of development of annulus fibrosus. Evidence of rudimentary joints, *A;* more normal apophyseal joints, *B.* Vertical measurement over the involved centra may distinguish this condition from fusion following infection; in malformations, this measure closely approximates that concerned with an equal number of normal bodies, whereas with destruction by infection, it is usually reduced. Note subnormal horizontal dimensions in **Figure 502 (right below).** **Figure 500 (right above)** shows not pathologic bridging but a developmental "block," localized at *C,* as indicated by abrupt delimitation of disk contour, *D.*

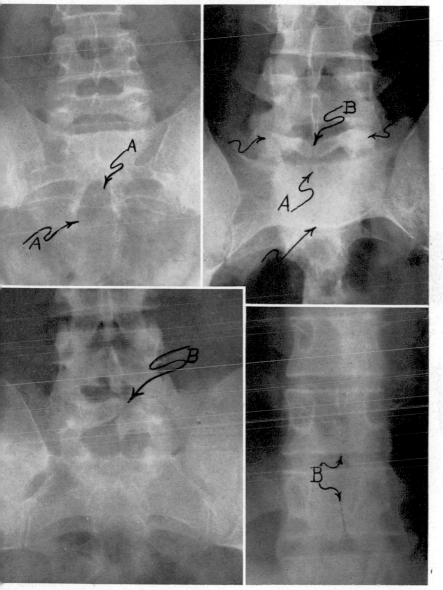

Figs. 503–506.—Failure of fusion of laminae is common, particularly in the lumbosacral region. There may be little or no formation of laminae, as in true spina bifida, A. Meningocele may complicate. Otherwise, laminae may be well formed and firmly support the meninges, as in spina bifida occulta, B. **Figure 504 (right above)** shows associated ossification defect in interarticular isthmi, as in spondylolisthesis, a not uncommon concomitant.

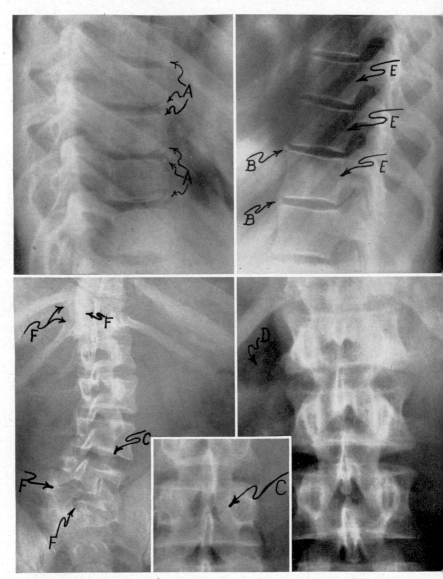

Figs. 507–511.—Secondary centers of ossification usually appear from 12 to 20. Developing epiphyses, A, must not be misinterpreted as fragmentations or osteochondropathic changes. Ununited ossifications between centra may be of the nature of a limbus vertebra, B—of no pathologic significance. Ununited epiphyses of articular processes, C, may be confusing when fracture is suspected; those of transverse processes, D, may simulate urinary calculi. Note nutrient artery grooves, E, and wedge-shaped centra, F.

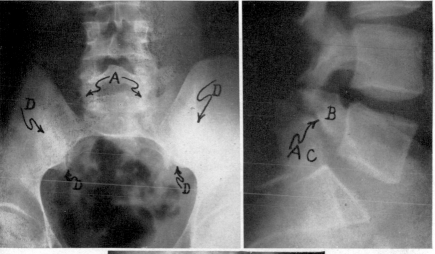

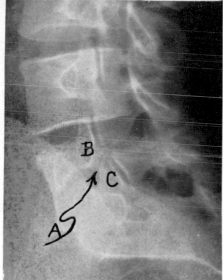

Figs. 512-514.—Defective ossification at isthmus, *A* —failure of union of superior, *B,* and inferior articular process, *C,* occurring in 3 to 5 per cent of persons. If there is no anterior slipping of upper portion of the spine, it is described as prespondylolisthesis or spondylolysis. Note visualization of the defect in the oblique projection **(Fig. 514, below)** and osteosclerosis and spur formations around the sacro-iliac joints, *D* **(Fig. 512, left above).**

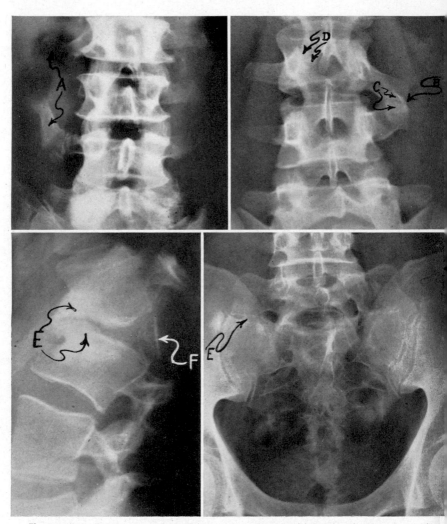

Fig. 523 (left above).—Anomalous rib formations, A. **Fig. 524 (right above).**—Articulation of transverse processes, B; note evidence of eburnation, C, signifying irritation and, doubtless, backache; ununited epiphysis, D, to be distinguished from fragmentation. **Fig. 525 (left below).**—Eburnations, E, attributable to hemivertebrae, F. **Fig. 526 (right below).**—Similar eburnation in case of overdeveloped transverse process of a lumbar vertebra (sacralization) or lack of synchondrosis of sacral segment (lumbarization).

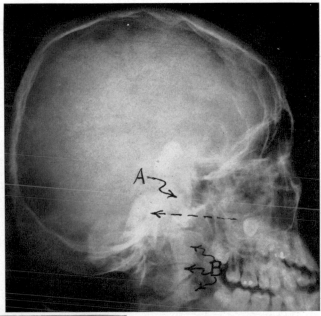

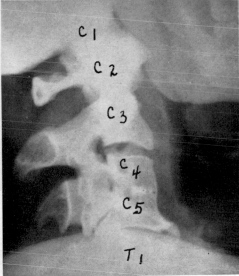

Fig. 527 (above).—Developmental protrusion of cervical spine into skull (basilar impression or platybasia). Note position of odontoid process, *A,* its extension above the line drawn from the hard palate to the posterior rim of the foramen magnum, causing short-necked appearance and possibly neuritic symptoms; malformations of centra, *B.* **Fig. 528 (left).**—Another condition possibly responsible for these features—block vertebra formations with only five segments (Klippel-Feil syndrome).

Spinal Osteochondropathies

SYNONYMS: When involvement is essentially of primary centers of ossification of centra: chronic vertebral rheumatism, kyphosis dorsalis juvenilis, osteochondritis juvenilis deformans, vertebra plana, kyphosis juvenilis, osteochondritis of the primary centers of the centra, Calvé's disease of the spine. When involvement is essentially concerned with secondary centers of ossification of centra—the epiphyses: vertebral epiphysitis, kyphosis adolescentium, Scheuermann's disease.

ROENTGEN CRITERIA

EARLY STAGES

Apophyseal joints: Likely, normal.

Amphi-arthrodial joints: Centra—irregularities; dissolutions and, possibly, actual erosions of osseous articular cortexes; possibly, fragmentations. (In case of involvement of primary centers of ossification, these changes are essentially concerned with middle portions of the centra; with involvement of secondary centers of ossification—the epiphysis—the changes are in anterior aspects of centra). Articular disks—apparent increase in interosseous spacing.

LATER STAGES

Apophyseal joints: Possibly, slight malalinement; eburnations of osseous articular cortexes; reduction of spacing between facets.

Amphi-arthrodial joints: Centra—osteosclerosis, especially bordering intra-osseous herniations of nucleus pulposus (Schmorl's nodes); likely, wedge-shaped compressions or actual flattenings even to wafer thinness, with increase on horizontal dimensions (platyspondyly); eburnations outlining erosions of osseous articular cortex; possibly, flattenings and spur formations. Articular disks—usually, spared, with little or no reduction in vertical dimensions; possibly, calcifications of nucleus pulposus.

Irregularities of alinement: Frequently, kyphosis; possibly, scoliosis.

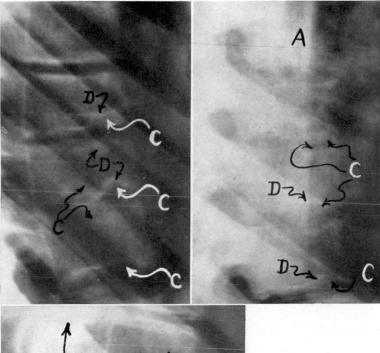

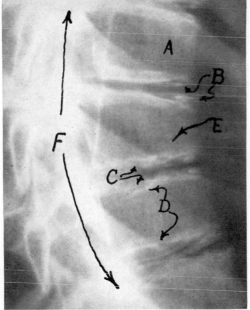

Figs. 529–531.—Relatively early stages of bone-cartilage pathology involving, essentially, primary centers. In **Figure 529 (left above),** ossification is not yet evident in secondary centers. Otherwise, note normal configuration of primary ossification, *A;* normal secondary ossification, *B;* irregular ossification and actual dissolution of osseous articular cortexes, *C;* regional osteosclerosis, *D;* anterior wedging in configuration of involved vertebrae, *E;* kyphosis, *F.*

CORROBORATIVE ROENTGEN CRITERIA: Possibly, evidence of old rickets elsewhere or endocrinopathy.

INCIDENCE

Age: Acute stage of involvement of primary centers of ossification usually before 10 years: for secondary centers (epiphyses of centra), 12–18 years.

Sex: Males more frequently involved.

Region: Usually, lower thoracic.

HISTORY: Insidious development of pain in lower thoracic or lumbar regions, with aggravation after exercise or with bending. At first, these may be interpreted as "growing pains"; later, they may prompt consideration of tuberculous spondylitis. Active children usually are concerned; ease of fatigability likely.

PHYSICAL FINDINGS: Usually general condition good; afebrile even during acute stages; likely, noticeable guarding of back, with rigid position in bed and resistance to movement; possibly, conspicuous kyphosis or scoliosis; possibly, palpable muscle spasm and tenderness on digital pressure around involved vertebrae.

LABORATORY FINDINGS: Usually noninformative.

CLINICAL COURSE: Alleviation of acute symptoms with bed rest for four to six months; later, deformity of posture; possibly, superimposed manifestations of osteo-arthropathy.

BIBLIOGRAPHY

BUCHMAN, J.: Osteochondritis of Vertebral Body, J. Bone & Joint Surg. 9:55–66, 1927.

CALVÉ, J.: Localized Affection of Spine Suggesting Osteochondritis of Vertebral Body, with Clinical Aspect of Pott's Disease, J. Bone & Joint Surg. 7:41–46, 1925.

KUHLMAN, F. Y.: Vertebra Plana (Calvé), Am. J. Roentgenol. 46:203–206, 1941.

NATHAN, L., AND KUHNS, J. G.: Epiphysitis of Spine, J. Bone & Joint Surg. 22:55–62, 1940.

SCHEUERMANN, H.: Scheuermann's Krankheit (Kyphosis Juvenilis), Fortschr. a.d. Geb. Röntgenstrahlen 53:1–16, 1936.

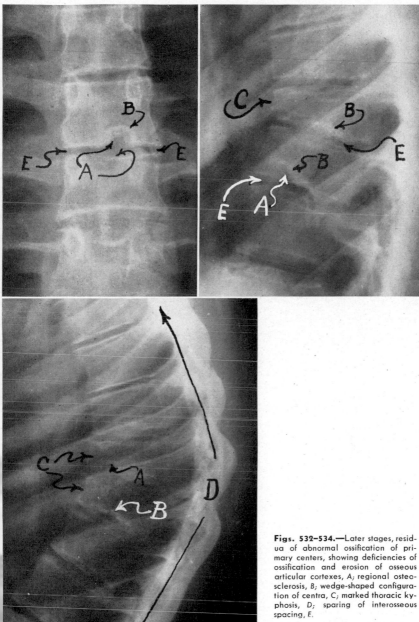

Figs. 532–534.—Later stages, residua of abnormal ossification of primary centers, showing deficiencies of ossification and erosion of osseous articular cortexes, *A;* regional osteosclerosis, *B;* wedge-shaped configuration of centra, *C;* marked thoracic kyphosis, *D;* sparing of interosseous spacing, *E.*

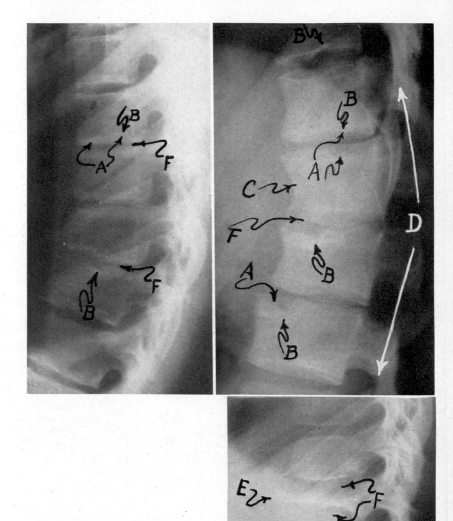

Figs. 535–537.—Various stages of spinal osteochondropathies concerned with primary centers. Irregularities and erosion of osseous articular cortexes, *A;* regional osteosclerosis, *B;* wedge-shaped deformation, *C;* kyphosis, *D;* actual flattening of body, *E;* sparing of interosseous spacing, *F.*

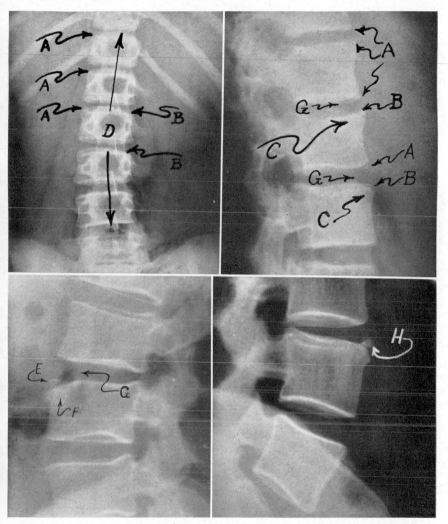

Figs. 538 and 539 (above).—Unilateral deficiencies in ossification of secondary centers. Normal epiphyseal development, *A;* deficient epiphyseal development, *B;* regional dissolution of primary ossifications, *C;* scoliosis, *D.* **Fig. 540 (left below).**—Residual evidence. Ununited secondary center of ossification, *E;.* osteosclerosis, *F;* sparing of interosseous spacing, *G.* **Fig. 541 (right below).**—Ununited epiphysis, *H,* with no evidence of dissolution or sclerosis of regional bone (a limbus vs. osteochondropathy).

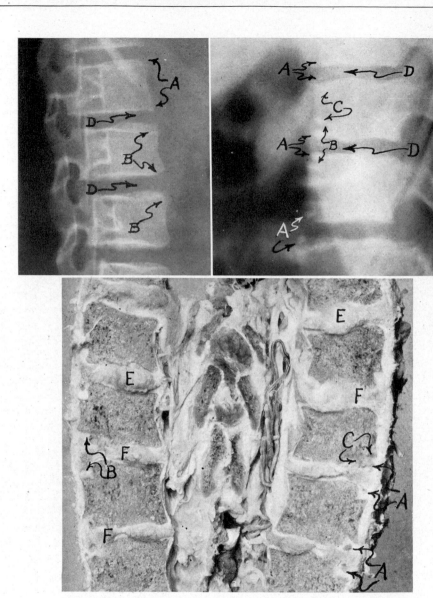

Fig. 542 (left above).—Early evidence of pathologic changes at sites of secondary ossification. **Fig. 543 (right above).**—Later stage. **Fig. 544 (below).**—Evidence at autopsy (death from other causes). Ununited centers (epiphyses), *A;* regional deossification and actual dissolution, *B;* osteosclerosis, *C;* sparing of interosseous spacing, *D.* In the longitudinal autopsy section, note expansion of normal nuclei pulposi, *E,* and apparent fibrotic changes of those near the osteochondropathic processes, *F.*

Spinal Osteo-Arthropathies: Traumatic

SYNONYMS: Discogenic disease, segmental neuritis, the radicular syndrome, degenerative disease of the spine, osteo-arthritis of the spine, spondylitis muscularis, cyphose heredo-traumatique, ankylosing spondylarthritis, spondylitis deformans, spondylosis ossificans, retropulsion of the intervertebral disk, prolapsed disk, herniation of the nucleus pulposus, Bechterew's spondylitis.

ROENTGEN CRITERIA

EARLY STAGES

Apophyseal joints: Roughening of osseous articular surfaces of facets; possibly, beginning eburnations; possibly, narrowing of interfacet spacing; possibly, partial subluxation or malalinements of articular processes.

Amphi-arthrodial joints: Centra—possibly, fracture line; likely, wedge-shaped deformation (anterior or lateral); possibly, eburnations; possibly, slight marginal lippings. Articular disks—likely, negative; possibly, slight reduction in intercentral spacing.

Curvatures: Possibly, malalinements of one or more centra with deviations from normal curvatures.

LATER STAGES

Apophyseal joints: Irregularities of alinement; eburnations and hypertrophic spurs or actual bridging across facets; possibly, osseous encroachments into root canals.

Amphi-arthrodial joints: Centra—possibly, wedge-shaped configurations (limited to one or few vertebrae); possibly, deossifications with coarsening of the trabeculation pattern; eburnations of articular cortexes; marginal spurs, lippings or actual intercentral bridging; possibly, erosions into cancellous structure (Schmorl's nodes). Articular disks—likely, irregular narrowings, especially of anterior portions.

Myelography: Air or opaque mediums injected into the canal may visualize a filling defect or perhaps failure of distribution of the medium around the nerve roots.

CORROBORATIVE ROENTGEN CRITERIA: Possibly, evidence of compression of vertebrae elsewhere or other evidence of traumatic arthropathies.

INCIDENCE

Age: Early changes during greatest physical activity; residua throughout life.

Sex: Males more frequently involved.

Sites of predilection: Eleventh or twelfth thoracic; first, second or fourth and fifth lumbars or fourth, fifth or sixth cervical.

HISTORY: Likely, background of trauma (e.g., a fall or automobile accident), with relief of immediate pain but months later development of tingling, drawing sensations or prickly and stinging "needle-like" irritations over the distribution of sciatic, brachial or any segmental nerve distribution with progressive increase in severity thereof. Pains likely aggravated by rising to sitting position or by sudden twists or other postures of strain to the spine; often pains are described as radiating "over the heart." Eventually, muscle spasm may be associated. Relief may be reported with flexion of the head, hence the tendency to use two or more pillows at night.

PHYSICAL FINDINGS: Alteration in normal curvatures; limitation in rotation movement; possibly, spasm or atrophy of muscle groups; hyper- or hypo-active reflexes; eliciting of areas of paresthesia or anesthesia or, possibly, actual paralysis; occasionally, psychic phenomona.

LABORATORY FINDINGS: Usually uninformative.

CLINICAL COURSE: Gradual but usually progressive increase in severity of symptoms and signs; possibly, intervals of freedom from them; possibly, alternation of sides of involvement. Because of the different positions of the root canals at the various levels, acute and progressive symptomatology is less likely to be associated with lesions in the thoracic region than with those in the cervical and lower lumbar regions.

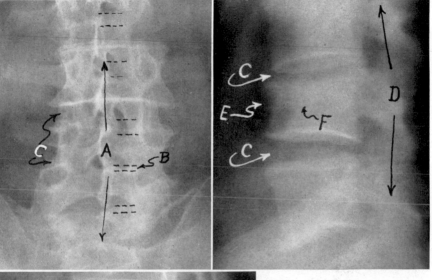

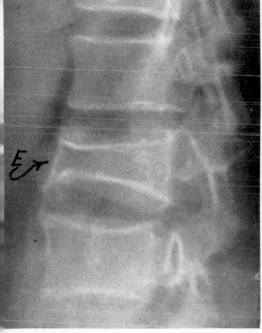

Figs. 545–547.—Violent vertical strain, as from a fall, usually damages midosseous structure rather than osseous articular cortexes or interosseous fibrocartilage. Owing to telescoping of fragments and leverage deviation of spinous processes, in addition to malalinement, A, A-P projection usually shows abrupt variation in interspacing of spinous processes, B, and, possibly, of centra, C. Lateral projections are usually more informative, perhaps showing kyphosis, D; wedge-shaped configuration, E; possibly, actual fracture line, F. First studies may be negative, yet 10–18 months later there may be evidence of marked absorption, with wedge-shaped deformity **(Fig. 547, left)** indicating old molecular fracture.

BIBLIOGRAPHY

BADGLEY, C. E.: Articular Facets in Relation to Low Back Pain and Sciatic Radiation, J. Bone & Joint Surg. 23:481–496, 1941.

BATTS, M., JR.: Rupture of Nucleus Pulposus: Anatomical Study, J. Bone & Joint Surg. 21:121–126, 1939.

BRAILSFORD, J. F.: Radiographic Investigation of Lumbar and Sciatic Pain, Brit. M. J. 2:827–830, 1932.

CHAMBERLAIN, W. E., AND YOUNG, B. R.: Air Myelography in Diagnosis of Intraspinal Lesions Producing Low Back and Sciatic Pain, Radiology 33:695–700, 1939.

DANDY, W. E.: Recent Advances in Diagnosis and Treatment of Ruptured Intervertebral Disks, Ann. Surg. 115:514–520, 1942.

GERIN, C.: Trauma ed artritismo apopisario del rachide [Relation of trauma to apophyseal arthritis in workmen: Medicolegal discussion], Arch. di antropol. crim. 53:1456–1466, 1933.

KELLY, L. C.: Chronic Hypertrophic Osteoarthritis in Cervical Spine with Radiculitis, New York State J. Med. 42:144, 1942.

METTIER, S. R., AND CAPP, C. S.: Neurological Symptoms and Clinical Findings in Patients with Cervical Degenerative Arthritis, Ann. Int. Med. 14:1315–1322, 1941.

MORTON, S. A.: Localized Hypertrophic Changes in Cervical Spine with Compression of Spinal Cord or of Its Roots, J. Bone & Joint Surg. 18:893–898, 1936.

OPPENHEIMER, A.: Apophyseal Intervertebral Joints, Surgery 8:699–712, 1940.

———, AND TURNER, E. L.: Discogenetic Disease of Cervical Spine with Segmental Neuritis, Am. J. Roentgenol. 37:484–493, 1937.

SEMMES, R. E., AND MURPHEY, F.: Intraspinal Rupture of Intervertebral Disc, J. Tennessee M. A. 35:49–52, 1942.

TURNER, E. L., AND OPPENHEIMER, A.: Common Lesion of Cervical Spine Responsible for Segmental Neuritis, Ann. Int. Med. 10:427–440, 1936.

WARTENBERG, R.: Myelography, J. Nerv. & Ment. Dis. 91:47–52, 1940.

WILLIAMS, P. C.: Reduced Lumbosacral Joint Space: Its Relation to Sciatic Irritation, J. A. M. A. 99:1677–1682, 1932.

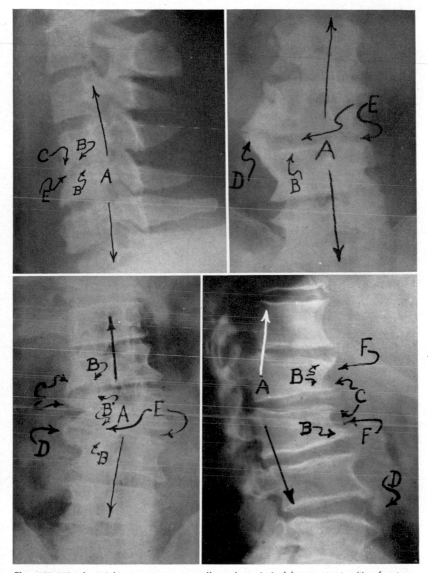

Figs. 548–551.—Less violent trauma may eventually produce principal damage at extremities of centra—osseous articular cortexes and fibrocartilaginous disks. This may be manifested by malalinement, *A* (emphasizing asymmetrical involvement); eburnation, *B;* marginal spurs, *C;* possibly, intercentral bridging, *D;* asymmetrical reduction of intercentral spacing, *E.* Wedge-shaped deformation, *F,* found after violent trauma, may also be present.

Spinal Osteo-Arthropathies: Static

SYNONYMS: Hypertrophic spondylitis, degenerative disease of the spine, osteo-arthritis of the spine, ankylosing spondylarthritis, spondylosis ossificans, Bechterew's spondylitis.

ROENTGEN CRITERIA

EARLY STAGES

Apophyseal joints: Beginning eburnations; irregularities of the facets; perhaps, marginal spurs; perhaps, reduction of interfacet spacings.

Amphi-arthrodial joints: Centra—coarsening of trabeculations; eburnations of osseous articular cortexes; marginal spurs. Articular disks—possibly, slight reduction of intercentral spacing.

Involvement of a *series* of vertebrae (rather than an isolated one or two): possibly, malalinements and resulting deviations from normal curvatures.

LATER STAGES

Apophyseal joints: Eburnations, roughening of facets; marginal spurs; reduction or obliteration of interfacet spacing.

Amphi-arthrodial joints: Centra—coarsening of trabeculation pattern; possibly, deossifications; flattenings; eburnations of osseous articular cortexes; marginal spurs; possibly, intercentral beakings; possibly, intercentral bridgings. Articular disks—asymmetrical reductions of interosseous spacing; possibly, calcifications of nucleus pulposus.

Involvement of series of vertebrae (rather than an isolated one or two): likely, kyphosis or other deviations from normal curvatures.

CORROBORATIVE ROENTGEN CRITERIA: Likely, evidence of osteo-arthropathies in other weight-bearing joints; possibly, evidence of developmental malformations, osteochondropathies, neuropathology, obesity or infections.

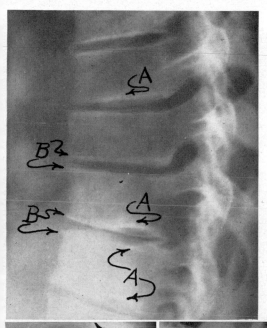

Figs. 565-568. — Static spinal osteo-arthropathies are characterized by early involvement of thoracic region and continuity of pathology with involvement of many vertebrae, with eburnations, A; marginal spurs, B (pertaining to osseous articular cortexes of both centra and apophyseal joints); intercentral bridging, C; kyphosis, D; wedge-shaped deformities, E.

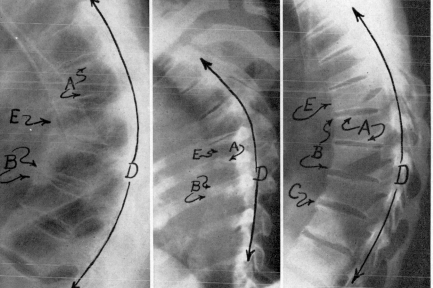

INCIDENCE

Age: Early stages, 25–40; residua throughout life.

Sex: Males more frequently involved.

Occupation: Arduous type, particularly requiring activity in abnormal positions.

HISTORY: Likely, arduous occupation requiring abnormal posture; otherwise, abnormal weight-bearing from other causes, including obesity; gradual development of backache; possibly, radiating pains, usually aggravated by sudden twisting or jerks.

PHYSICAL FINDINGS: Usually, healthy appearing individual; no evidence of sepsis; possibly, abnormalities of posture and curvatures; limitations of movement of spine; possibly, tenderness on digital pressure at various levels.

LABORATORY FINDINGS: Likely, irrelevant.

CLINICAL COURSE: Usually, progressive increase in severity of aching; limitation of movements regardless of intervals of alleviation.

BIBLIOGRAPHY

DAWSON, M. H.: Osteoarthritis of Spine, J. Lab. & Clin. Med. 22:25, 1936.

DOUB, H. P.: Chronic Arthritis of Spine, Radiology 22:147–152, 1934.

GILLESPIE, J.: Case of Arthritis of Spine with Neurological Manifestations, Irish J. M. Sc., pp. 215–219, 1937.

GUNTHER, L.: Pain of Nerve Root Origin in Hypertrophic Osteoarthritis of Spine As Confusing Factor in Diagnosis, J. Lab. & Clin. Med. 15:1257–1264, 1930.

———, AND KERR, W. J.: Radicular Syndrome in Hypertrophic Osteo-Arthritis of Spine, Arch. Int. Med. 43:212–248, 1929.

HAMPTON, A. O., AND ROBINSON, J. M.: Roentgenographic Demonstration of Rupture of Intervertebral Disc into Spinal Canal after Injection of Lipiodol, with Special Reference to Unilateral Lumbar Lesions Accompanied by Low Back Pain with "Sciatic" Radiation, Am. J. Roentgenol. 36:782–803, 1936.

LUX, A.: Spondylarthritis Due to Posture and Its Treatment, Am. J. Surg. 48:654–657, 1940.

MACGOWAN, T. J. B. A.: Examination of Normal and Adolescent Kyphotic Spines, Glasgow M. J. 133:206–209, 1940.

ZABRISKIE, E. G.; HARE, C. C., AND MASSELINK, R. J.: Hypertrophic Arthritis of Cervical Vertebrae with Thenar Muscular Atrophy Occurring in Three Sisters, Bull. Neurol. Inst., New York 4:207–220, 1935.

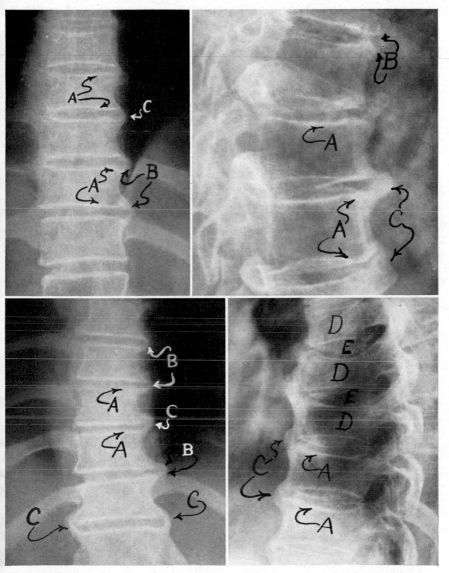

Figs. 569–572.—After prolonged strain, the changes extend downward, involving larger and larger vertebrae. Eburnations, *A*, become more marked. Marginal spurs, *B*, become continuous, forming beakings or bridgings, *C*. Many of these are misinterpreted as calcifications in ligaments and therefore diagnosed descending rheumatoid (Marie-Strümpell's) spondylitis. As in the latter condition, there may be deossification (secondarily), *D*; biconcave deformations of vertebrae owing to expansion of nucleus pulposus, *E*.

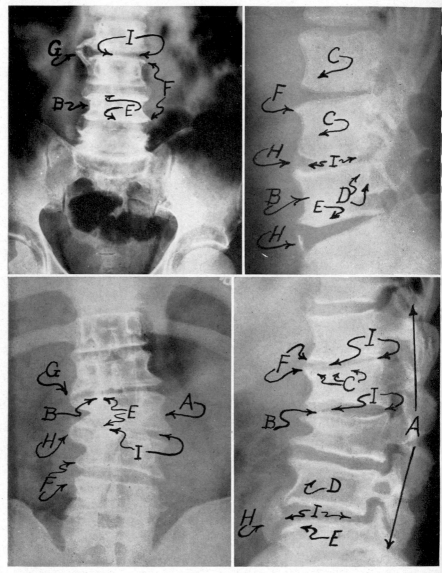

Figs. 573–576.—Strenuous physical activity in abnormal positions, as in mining, may cause marked changes with involvement of a series of vertebrae, including both thoracic and lumbar; malalinement, *A*; flattening, *B*; cystic deossification, *C*; coarsening of trabeculations, *D*; eburnation of osseous articular cortexes, *E*; marginal spurs, *F*; intercentral beaking, *G*; intercentral bridging, *H*; asymmetrical reduction of intercentral spacing, *I*.

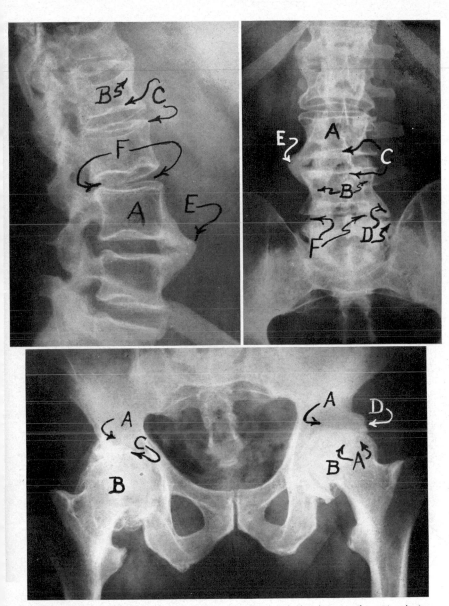

Figs. 577–579.—Changes similar to those in Figures 573–576 may be found in cases of excessive obesity with concurrent inactivity. Seemingly, inactivity results in deossification, *A;* the weight strain causing coarsening of trabeculations, *B;* eburnation, *C;* marginal spurs, *D;* intercentral beaking, *E;* asymmetrical intercentral spacing, *F.* In such cases, these changes are likely to be found not only in the spine but in weight-bearing joints such as the hips **(Fig. 579, below).** Note bilaterality.

Spinal Osteo-Arthropathy: Senescent

SYNONYMS: Senile spondyl-osteo-arthropathy, senile osteoporosis, postmenopausal spondylitis, atrophy of disuse, abiotrophy, degenerative spondylitis.

ROENTGEN CRITERIA

EARLY STAGES

Apophyseal joints: Deossification of articular processes; thinning of osseous articular cortexes; irregularities of facets; slight spur formations.

Amphi-arthrodial joints: Centra—deossification with thinning of trabeculations and *increased* spacing between them; slight eburnation of osseous articular cortexes; slight spur formations. Articular disks—likely, expanded; possibly, intracentral extrusions (Schmorl's nodes).

LATER STAGES

Apophyseal joints: Deossifications; possibly, fusion of facets; possibly, malappositions.

Amphi-arthrodial joints: Centra—marked deossification; biconcavities of configuration; possibly, compressions or telescopic fractures; slight eburnations; slight lipping. Articular disks—likely, expanded; possibly, calcified; possibly, malalinements with accentuation or flattening of normal curvature.

CORROBORATIVE ROENTGEN CRITERIA: Evidence of senescent osteo-arthropathies of the extremities.

INCIDENCE

Age: Past 40.

Sex: Females more frequently involved (three or four to one male).

HISTORY: Inactivity for years; gradual development of backache with intermittent disturbance; possibly, abrupt development of acute pains (due to fracture); occasionally, notice of reduction in stature.

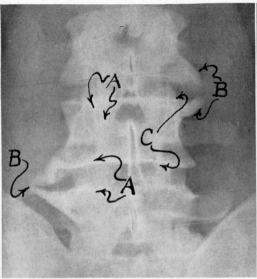

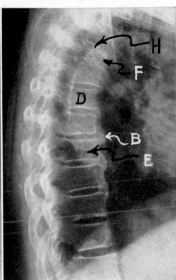

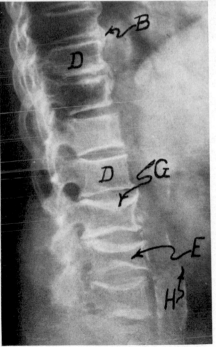

Figs. 580–582.—In persons past 40, there may be residual changes concerned with factors other than senescence, particularly those attributable to repeated stresses of weight-bearing: eburnation, *A;* marginal spurs, beaking or bridging, *B;* possibly, slight irregularity of osseous articular cortexes, *C.* More specifically, this age group shows signs of inactivity: deossification, *D;* flattening or compression, *E;* possibly, actual fracture, *F,* and intracentral intrusion of the nucleus pulposus with concavities or actual node formation, *G.* Note calcific streaking outlining the aorta, *H.*

PHYSICAL FINDINGS: Elderly appearing, nontoxic individual manifesting slight guarding of back; likely, some abnormality of curvature; possibly, tenderness on digital pressure.

LABORATORY FINDINGS: Likely, uninformative.

CLINICAL COURSE: Usually progressive; increase in symptoms with repeated fractures.

BIBLIOGRAPHY

ALBERT, M.: Calcification of Intervertebral Disks, Brit. M. J. 1:666–668, 1942.
BÁRSONY, T., AND POLGÁR, F.: Calcinosis Intervertebralis, Klin. Wchnschr. 4:759, 1925.
Cabot Case 25161: Gout: Hypertrophic (Degenerative) Arthritis of Spine, New England J. Med. 220:676–684, 1939.
DARLEY, W.; GORDON, R. W., AND MATCHETT, F.: Spontaneous Vertebral Compression Fractures Due to Senile Osteoporosis, Rocky Mountain M. J. 39:193–196, 1942.
LANCE, M.; GIRARD, L., AND LANCE, P.: Les ostéoporoses et malacies du rachis chez l'adult [Osteoporosis and osteomalacia in adults, especially in old age], Rev. d'orthop. 25:385–448, 1938.
NATHANSON, L., AND LEWITAN, A.: Deformities and Fractures of Vertebrae As Result of Senile and Presenile Osteoporosis, Am. J. Roentgenol. 46:197–202, 1941.
ZACHO, A.: Osteoporosis and Osteomalacia Columnae, Acta orthop. Scandinav. 11:264–295, 1940.

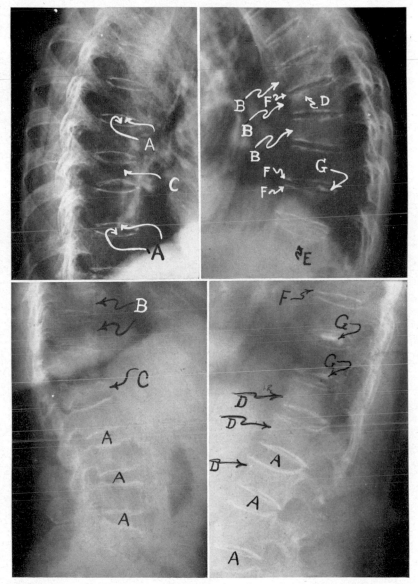

Figs. 583–586.—Changes associated with deossification may be so marked as to simulate hyperparathyroidism or early stage of plasma cell myeloma. Concavities in configuration of centra, A; multiplicity of wedge-shaped vertebrae, B; compressions, C; actual fractures, D; intracentral extrusions of nucleus pulposus, E. Marginal lipping or spur formations, F, may be inconspicuous. Note calcification of nucleus pulposus, G in **Figures 584 (right above) and 586 (right below).**

Spinal Neuro-Arthropathies: Simple

SYNONYMS: Motor nerve paralysis of spinal musculature, spine of poliomyelitis, neuratrophic spine, Heine-Medin's disease of spine.

ROENTGEN CRITERIA:

EARLY STAGES

Apophyseal joints: Serial derangements of alinement of articular processes; slight eburnations of osseous articular cortexes; irregularities of facets.

Amphi-arthrodial joints: Centra—deossifications with thinning of trabeculations; slight eburnations. Articular disks—asymmetrical spacings.

Malalinements: Scoliosis; kyphosis.

LATER STAGES

Apophyseal joints: Derangements of alinement of articular processes; deossifications; eburnations; reduction in interspacing between facets; possibly, fibrous ankylosis.

Amphi-arthrodial joints: Centra—conspicuous deossifications; slight eburnations; marginal lippings; possibly, wedge-shaped compressions. Articular disks—asymmetrical reductions in vertical dimensions.

Malalinements: Scoliosis; kyphosis.

CORROBORATIVE ROENTGEN CRITERIA: Asymmetrical contraction of thorax; possibly, eventration of diaphragm; possibly, evidence of simple neuro-arthropathic changes of peripheral joints.

CLINICAL AND LABORATORY FINDINGS: Same as those in similar conditions of peripheral joints.

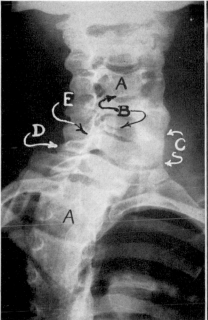

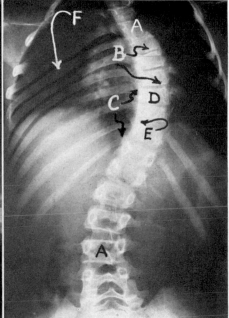

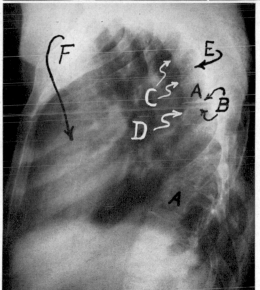

Lesions of anterior horns or efferent nerves may produce such atrophy of muscle groups as to cause imbalance of opposing spinal supports and thereby scoliosis **(Figs. 587 and 588, above)** and possibly kyphosis **(Fig. 589, left).** This explanation of such deformities should be considered after making certain that there are no developmental anomalies or infectious spondylitis, these two possibilities being more common. Otherwise, criteria of importance include: slender trabeculation pattern, A (due to limited use); slight eburnation, B (even in the young); marginal lipping, C; wedge-shaped deformation, D; possibly, reduction of intercentral spacing, E. Contraction of thoracic cage, F, can be expected.

Spinal Neuro-Arthropathies:
Charcot Type

SYNONYMS: Sensory nerve paralysis of spinal musculature, tabetic spondylitis, syphilitic spondylitis, spondylitis of tabes dorsalis, spondylitis of dorsal column damage.

ROENTGEN CRITERIA

EARLY STAGES

Apophyseal joints: Derangements of alinement of one or a few articular processes; eburnations of osseous articular cortexes; marginal spurs.

Amphi-arthrodial joints: Centra—eburnations of osseous articular cortexes; marginal spurs; possibly, intercentral bridgings. Articular disks—asymmetrical reductions in vertical dimensions.

Localized malalinements: Abrupt scoliosis, kyphosis or lordosis.

LATER STAGES

Apophyseal joints: Malalinements of articular processes; marked eburnations; spur formations; bridgings; possibly, fragmentations.

Amphi-arthrodial joints: Centra—eburnations; marginal spurs; intercentral bridgings; fragmentations of osseous articular cortexes and bodies. Articular disks—asymmetrical obliterations.

Localized malalinements: Abrupt scoliosis, kyphosis or lordosis; lower lumbar and upper sacral vertebrae most severely involved.

CORROBORATIVE ROENTGEN CRITERIA: Possibly, evidence of similar changes in most active weight-bearing joints: ankles, knees or hips; possibly, evidence of syphilitic heart disease.

CLINICAL AND LABORATORY FINDINGS: Same as those found in similar conditions of peripheral joints.

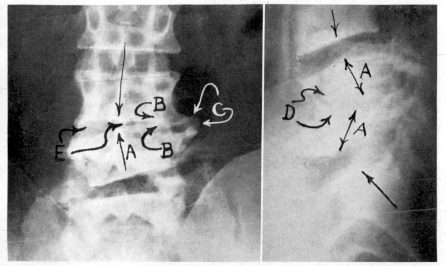

Figs. 590 and 591.—Loss of function of posterior horns or afferent nerves may result in such abnormalities of weight carriage as to produce malalinement of one or more centra, A; eburnation of osseous articular cortexes, B; marginal spurs, C; fragmentation of osseous articular cortexes, D; asymmetrical obliteration of intercentral disks, E.

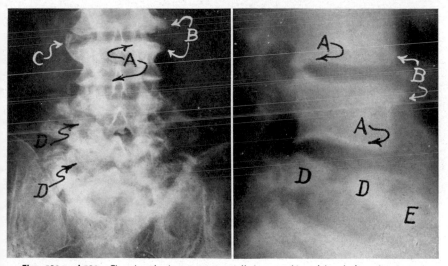

Figs. 592 and 593.—Though early changes are essentially hypertrophic and though eburnation, A, marginal spurs, B, and intercentral bridging, C, may be found, continued excessive punishment of lower lumbar vertebrae produces fragmentation of bones, D. Because of continued use, there being lack of sensory inhibition, appearance may be that of sclerotic débris, E.

Spinal Rheumatoid Arthritis

SYNONYMS: Rheumatoid arthritis of the spine, atrophic spondylitis, Marie-Strümpell's disease, chronic ankylosing spondylitis, spondylitis ossificans ligamentosa, spondylitis deformans, spondylarthritis ankylopoietica, spondylitis chronica ankylopoietica, spondylitis rhizomélique, inflammatory spondylitis, poker spine, bamboo spine, ankylosing spondylarthritis.

ROENTGEN CRITERIA

EARLY STAGES

Apophyseal joints: Deossification of articular processes; narrowing of interfacet spacing; irregularities of facets.

Sacro-iliac joints: Marginal decalcification and mottling (bilaterally).

Amphi-arthrodial joints: Centra—blurring of osseous articular cortexes. Articular disks—likely, normal.

Flattening of lordotic curvature.

LATER STAGES

Apophyseal joints: Calcific streaking (syndesmophytes) or actual bridging along ligamentum flavum; fixation of joints.

Sacro-iliac joints: Obliteration by actual bridging.

Amphi-arthrodial joints: Centra—deossifications; calcific streaking or actual bridging in anterior paraspinal ligament and, finally, in posterior paraspinal ligament. Articular disks—seldom reduction in vertical dimensions; possibly, expansions; seldom, roughening in the articular surfaces of centra; tendency toward biconvex configuration (i.e., concave articular surfaces so far as centra are concerned).

Exaggeration of thoracic kyphosis, regardless of flattening of lumbar lordosis; flattening of cervical lordosis.

CORROBORATIVE ROENTGEN CRITERIA: Progressive extension of pathologic changes from lumbosacral region *upward;*

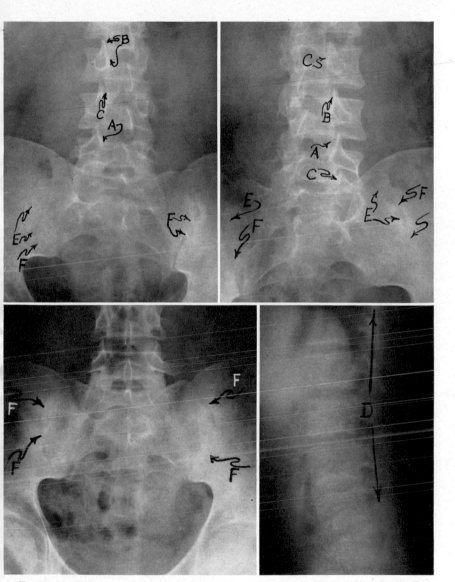

Figs. 594–597.—Roentgen manifestations during earliest phases may be limited to deossification of osseous articular cortexes of apophyseal joints, *A*; reduction of spacing between facets, *B*; obliteration, *C*. With these are flattening of lumbar lordosis, *D*, and concurrently or soon thereafter, mottled deossification along sacro-iliac joints, *E*, with progressive obliteration, *F*.

ultimate fixation of costovertebral joints and limitation of thoracic excursions; possibly, evidence of foci of infection; frequently, evidence of atrophic arthritis elsewhere (especially, hips and shoulders); possibly, associated lithiasis of urinary tract.

INCIDENCE

Age: Medical attention usually sought between 20 and 40; acute symptomatology may date back to childhood.

Sex: Approximately 90 per cent males.

Habits: Usually, sedentary.

HISTORY: Usually, vague low back pain; possibly, bouts of acute sciatica; possibly, radiating pains in chest or abdomen; (pleurodynia, kidney or intestinal disturbances, muscular rheumatism, etc.); frequently, attacks of genito-urinary infection ("60 per cent"—Forestier), including gonorrhea; possibly, pulmonary tuberculosis, iritis or pneumonia; loss of weight; progressive weakness; progressive stiffness of the back.

PHYSICAL FINDINGS: Usually, a slender, cold, clammy and emaciated type of individual, guarding in rotation movements and bending, bearing a rigid posture, with shallow chest and ptotic abdomen; head and shoulders bent forward, likely showing diminished thoracic excursions; possibly, complaining of tenderness on digital pressure over sacro-iliac regions, spinous processes or apophyseal joints; possibly, fusiform swellings around joints of extremities and stiffness or actual ankylosis of these, as well as rigidity of the spinal column; possibly, spasms of dorsal muscles and atrophy in dorsolumbar region; hyperesthesia; possibly, low grade fever; frequently, iritis.

LABORATORY FINDINGS: Accelerated sedimentation rate (during stage of inflammatory activity); abnormally high flocculation (resorcin test of Vernes); likely, mild microcytic anemia; possibly, leukocytosis.

CLINICAL COURSE: Usually, progressive fixation of joints with thoracic kyphosis; favorable response to colloidal gold therapy or small doses of roentgen rays.

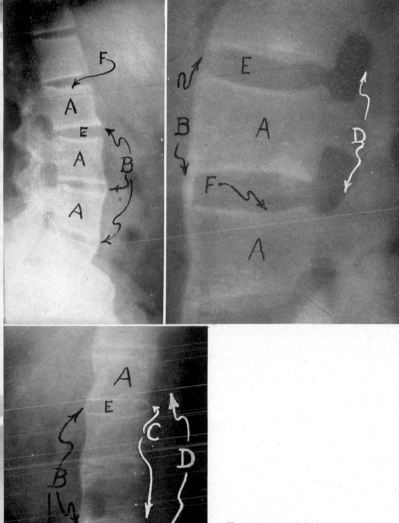

Figs. 598–600.—With progression, there may be deossification, *A;* calcification of anterior spinal ligament, *B,* and eventually also of posterior spinal ligament, *C,* and ligamentum flavum, *D.* Usually intercentral spacing is unchanged, *E;* or, owing to deossification and pressure of nucleus pulposus, there may be actual expansion of the disk, *F.* These changes usually extend from the lumbosacral region upward.

BIBLIOGRAPHY

BAKER, L. D.: Rhizomelic Spondylitis; Orthopaedic and Roentgen Therapy, J. Bone & Joint Surg. 24:827–830, 1942.

BLAIR, H. C.: Spondylitis Adolescens—Struempell-Marie Disease; Practical and Theoretical Considerations, Surg., Gynec. & Obst. 74:663–670, 1942.

BUCHMANN, E.: Spondylitis Ankylopoietica, Nord. med. 5:12–20, 1940.

EDSTRÖM, G.: Is Spondylarthritis Ankylopoietica Independent Disease or Rheumatic Syndrome? Acta med. Scandinav. 104:396–413, 1940.

FORESTIER, J.: Importance of Sacro-Iliac Changes in Early Diagnosis of Ankylosing Spondylarthritis, Marie-Strümpell-Bechterew Disease, Radiology 33:389–402, 1939.

FREUND, E.: Contribution to Pathogenesis of Spondylitis Ankylopoietica, Edinburgh M. J. 49:91–109, 1942.

HALL, E. W.: Ankylosing Spondylitis and Polyarthritis (Bechterew, Strümpell-Marie and Related Types), Am. J. Roentgenol. 30:608–614, 1933.

HARE, H. F.: Diagnosis of Marie-Strümpell Arthritis with Certain Aspects of Treatment, New England J. Med. 223:702–705, 1940.

KNAGGS, R. L.: Spondylitis Deformans, Brit. J. Surg. 12:524–546, 1925.

LASSEN, N.: Early Diagnosis of Spondylarthritis Ankylopoietica, Ugesk f. laeger 101:1307–1312, 1939.

MARIE, P.: Sur la spondylose rhizomélique [On rhizomelic spondylosis], Rev. de méd. 18:285–345, 1898.

MILLER, J. L.: Differential Diagnosis between Strümpell-Marie Disease and Osteoarthritis of Spine, J. Lab. & Clin. Med. 22:19–22, 1936.

TYSON, T. L.: Spondylitis Ankylopoietica, M. Clin. North America 21:1755–1761, 1937.

VONTZ, O.: Röntgendiagnostik der Spondylarthritis ancylopoetica (Bechterew) [Roentgen diagnosis of spondylarthritis ankylopoietica (Bechterew's disease)], Deutsche med. Wchnschr. 63:1558–1559, 1937.

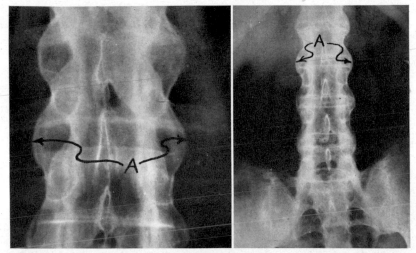

Figs. 601 and 602.—Later, intervertebral ligaments (annulus fibrosus) show calcification peripherally, A, developing thereby a "bamboo" configuration. Intercentral spacing remains normal or is increased.

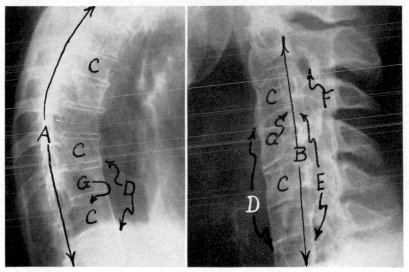

Figs. 603 and 604.—Thoracic and cervical portions may later be involved. Normal thoracic kyphosis becomes exaggerated, A, while normal cervical lordosis becomes flattened, B. Otherwise, features are: deossification, C; calcification, first of anterior spinal ligament, D, and later of posterior spinal ligament, E, and ligamentum flavum, F. Disks retain normal dimensions or become expanded, G.

disks—reduction of vertical dimension (usually symmetrical); possibly, intercentral fusions (i.e., ankylosis—osseous in children, likely fibrous with cleavage line in adults).

Abrupt malalinements: Especially, kyphosis; possibly, scoliosis.

CORROBORATIVE ROENTGEN CRITERIA: Likely, positive findings in chest (particularly pneumonic consolidations, recent or remote) or genito-urinary tract. Usually, processes in spine *isolated* rather than of serial sequence; possibly, one or two joints concerned with one process, another one or two at a distant level. Possibly, evidence of bone or joint lesions elsewhere (50 per cent of tuberculous involvement of bone occurs in spine).

INCIDENCE

Age: Usually early childhood, 2–6; adolescence, 12–16, or early adult life.

Sex: Irrelevant.

Race: More common and more severe among colored race.

HISTORY: Likely, background of acute illness (mere lassitude, fever and malaise of primary phase of tuberculosis or more clinically evident respiratory symptomatology of reinfection phase of tuberculosis or the acute manifestations of a true pneumonic process such as produced by staphylococcus, brucella, etc., or perhaps symptoms of typhoid fever); perhaps, alleviation of such signs and thereafter sudden exacerbation of chills, fever and toxicity with extreme aching in spine; limitation and pain on motion.

PHYSICAL FINDINGS: During earlier stages, patient usually toxic with septic type of fever; pulse and respiration variable. Posture usually rigid; possibly, conspicuous kyphosis or scoliosis with tenderness on digital pressure over spinous processes at levels of greatest deviation; likely, palpable muscle spasms; possibly, palpable intra-abdominal, intrapelvic or subinguinal masses; possibly, sinus drainage to back or inguinal region.

LABORATORY FINDINGS

Blood: Red cells possibly reduced to 2,500,000 or 3,000,000. Hemoglobin likely reduced to 70 per cent or less. White cells likely re-

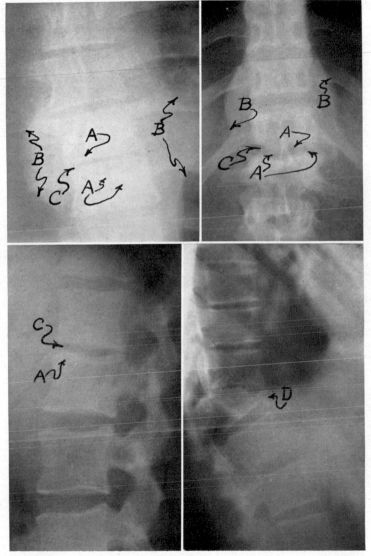

Figs. 608–611.—Progressive stages. When organisms thrive, especially in portions of bone where hemopoiesis and red bone marrow are lacking, progressive destruction, *A*, occurs, with resulting extravasation of organisms into fibrocartilage between the centra and also peripherally, producing a paraspinal abscess, *B*. These changes are inconspicuous at first **(Fig. 610, left below).** Careful search should be made for them whenever there is reduction of intercentral spacing, *C*. Serial studies are likely to reveal definite destruction of bone and possibly compression fractures, *D* **(Fig. 611, right below,** is same case as **Fig. 610,** but five months later).

duced (tuberculosis, typhoid or brucellosis); usually, increased monocytic and lymphocytic proportions and actual counts. Sedimentation rate increased. Agglutination test possibly specific (brucella, B typhosus, etc.).

Skin tests: Likely positive to specific proteins, with associated flare-up of back pain.

CLINICAL COURSE: Variable, depending on organism; possibly, response to chemotherapy with alleviation of symptoms and reossification of involved bone; otherwise, prolonged incapacitation with definite requirement of bed rest and thereby gradual involution of the process over several years; thereafter, likely, ankylosis of affected one or few joints, with deformity of stature.

BIBLIOGRAPHY

BISHOP, W. A.: Vertebral Lesions in Undulant Fever, J. Bone & Joint Surg. 21:665–673, 1939.

BOWEN, A., AND McGEHEE, C. L.: Typhoid Spine, Radiology 27:357–358, 1936.

DOUB, H. P., AND BADGLEY, C. E.: Roentgen Signs of Tuberculosis of Vertebral Body, Am. J. Roentgenol. 27:827–834, 1932.

HARRIS, R. I., AND COULTHARD, M. S.: Early Diagnosis of Pott's Disease, Ann. Surg. 114:931–935, 1941.

KEY, J. A.: Pathology of Tuberculosis of the Spine, J. Bone & Joint Surg. 22:799–806, 1940.

KULOWSKI, J.: Undulant (Malta) Fever Osteomyelitis and Arthritis, Surg., Gynec. & Obst. 62:759–763, 1936.

————: Pyogenic Osteomyelitis of Spine; Analysis and Discussion of 102 Cases, J. Bone & Joint Surg. 18:343–364, 1936.

PERLMAN, R., AND FREIBERG, J. A.: Vertebral Bridging in Tuberculosis of Spine, J. Bone & Joint Surg. 25:340–350, 1943.

PHALEN, G. S.; PRICKMAN, L. E., AND KRUSEN, F. H.: Brucellosis Spondylitis: Treatment by Physically Induced Hyperpyrexia, J. A. M. A. 118:859–862, 1942.

TABB, J. L., AND TUCKER, J. T.: Actinomycosis of Spine, Am. J. Roentgenol. 29:628–634, 1933.

WESTERMARK, N., AND FORSSMAN, G.: Roentgen Diagnosis of Tuberculous Spondylitis, Acta radiol. 19:207–214, 1938.

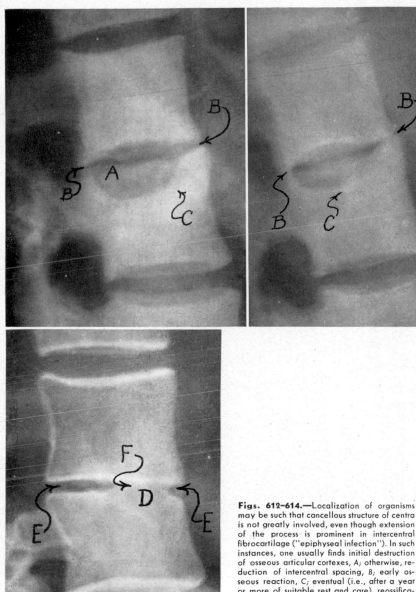

Figs. 612–614.—Localization of organisms may be such that cancellous structure of centra is not greatly involved, even though extension of the process is prominent in intercentral fibrocartilage ("epiphyseal infection"). In such instances, one usually finds initial destruction of osseous articular cortexes, *A;* otherwise, reduction of intercentral spacing, *B;* early osseous reaction, *C;* eventual (i.e., after a year or more of suitable rest and care), reossification, *D,* with residual reduction of intercentral spacing, *E,* and possibly intercentral fusion, *F.*

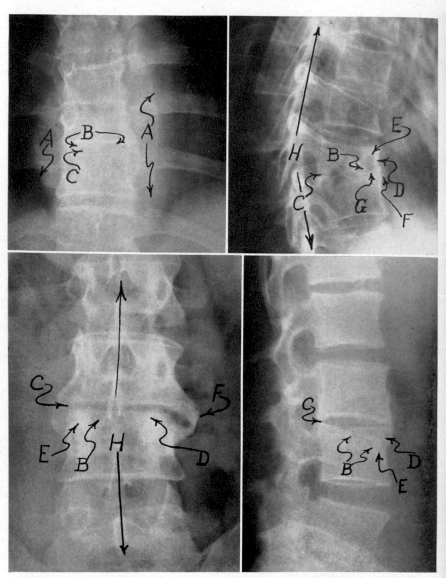

Figs. 615–618.—Soft tissue abscesses may extend along the longitudinal ligament and ultimately produce secondary processes. These figures all pertain to a single case. Note involvement of lower thoracic region (commonest location) and isolated involvement of third and fourth lumbars. Important criteria include: soft tissue tumefaction, *A;* bone destruction, *B;* reduction of intercentral spacing, *C;* compression, *D.* In addition, repair is evident: osteosclerosis, *E;* intercentral bridging, *F;* fusion, *G* (i.e., osseous ankylosis). Note also, deviations of alinement, *H.*

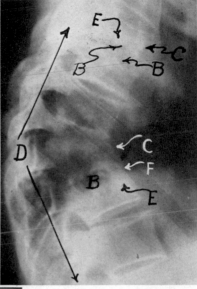

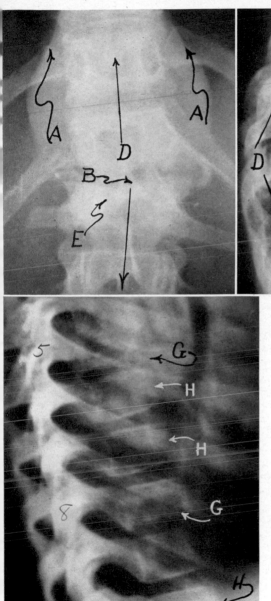

A soft tissue tumefaction, A, tapering upward suggests a process higher up. **Figures 619 and 620 (above)** pertain to the same case. Bone destruction, B; compressions, C; abrupt deviations of alinement, D. Evidence of healing includes osteosclerosis, E, and intercentral fusion, F. **Figure 621 (left)** shows multiplicity of localizations, G (and normal grooves for nutrient arteries, H).

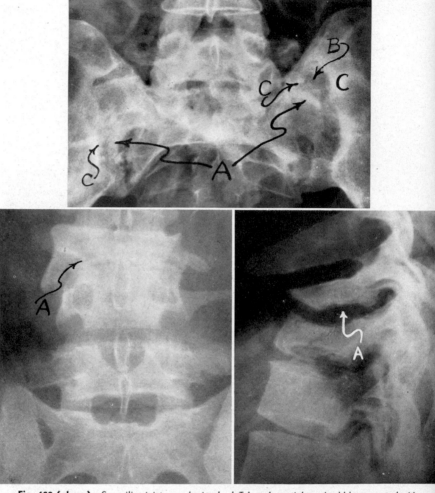

Fig. 622 (above).—Sacro-iliac joints may be involved. Tuberculous etiology should be suspected with bilateral involvement, A; marked destruction of bone, B; minimal osteosclerotic reaction, C, and corroborative evidence of a process higher up, with abrupt deviation of alinement. **Figs. 623 and 624 (below).**—Particularly with tuberculous infections, bone destruction may be extensive, involving half or more of a centrum (or appendage), A. In this respect, the Charcot type of spinal neuro-arthropathy may be simulated, though in infectious types, the thoracic or upper lumbar regions, rather than the lower lumbar or lumbosacral regions, are usually involved. Furthermore, sclerotic débris in the region of destruction is not usual in the infectious type; nor are marginal spurs or eburnations in centra above and below, as usually seen in the Charcot type. Patients' age may be distinctive, Charcot changes seldom being found in the young.

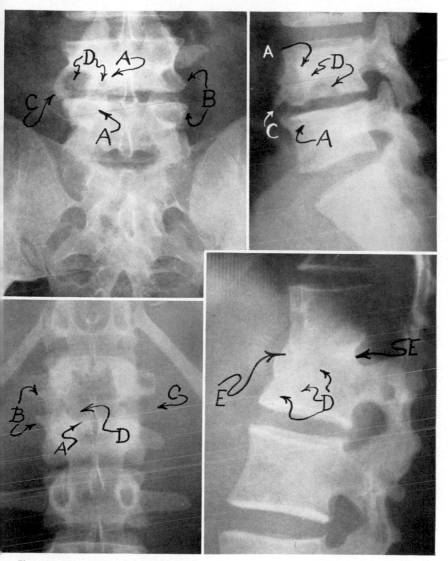

Figs. 625–628.—With involution of an infectious process, osteo-arthropathy of the post-traumatic type may be simulated because of osteosclerosis, A (simulating eburnations of post-traumatic type); marginal spurs, B; intercentral beaking, C. Localized involvement may be a feature of either, but evidence of bone destruction, D, and intercentral fusion, E, points to infectious etiology.

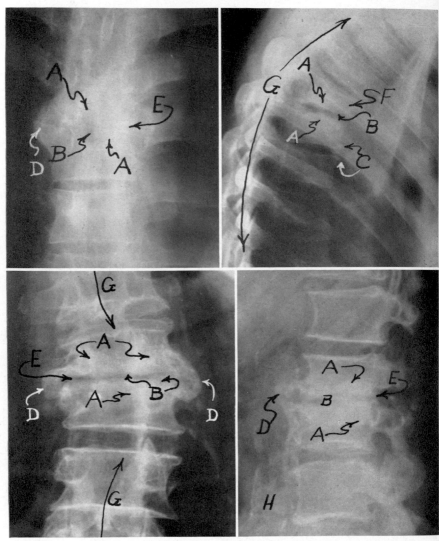

Figs. 629–632.—Infections with pyogenes such as staphylococci are usually characterized by less bone destruction in the main portions of bone than in infections with the tubercle bacillus, with more bone production, likely conspicuous osteosclerosis, A, not only in the region of articular cortexes but also at a distance, thus distinguishing the case as one of infection instead of osteo-arthropathy following local trauma. Otherwise, there may be destruction of osseous articular cortexes, B; marginal spurs, C; inter-central bridging, D; reduction of intercentral spacing, E; wedge-shaped deformations, F; abrupt malaline-ment, G. (Note calcification in aorta, H.)

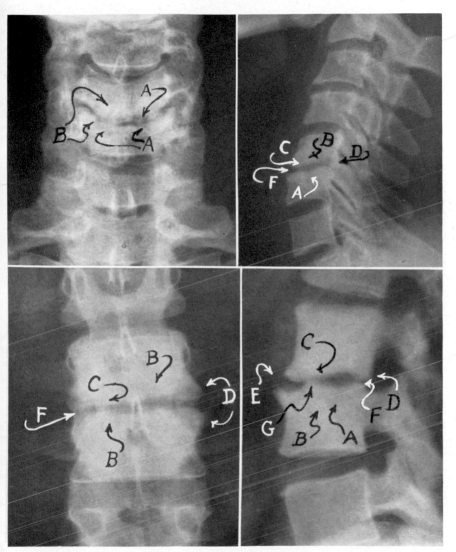

During scourges of typhoid fever, localization o that infection in the spine is not uncommon. Today, a more common etiologic factor is a brucella infection **(Figs. 633–636)**, with which the changes usually are those described for the pyogenic group: minimal bone destruction, A; conspicuous bone production, B; eburnation, C; marginal spurs, D; intercentral bridging, E; reduction of intercentral spacing, F; possibly, osseous ankylosis, G. Involvement of the bone proper should distinguish the infectious type from osteo-arthropathy.

Malformations of the vascular bed may occur. These may be of such dimensions as to warrant the description "hemangioma." As such, they may be identified as isolated regions of increased ray transparency, separated by partitions of markedly coarsened trabeculation structure. There may be evidence of diminished strength— even to the extent of flattening of the bone (especially in the case of the centrum) in the plane of weight support. There may also be evidence of intrusions of the nucleus pulposus.

Such lesions are to be distinguished from the more destructive and more multilocular defects produced by giant cell tumors. The importance of this distinction is concerned with treatment—the definite indication for roentgenotherapy in the case of giant cell tumors. With giant cell tumors, the bone destruction is much more conspicuous in any one location than with hemangiomas, and this destruction is likely to extend beyond the limits of any one portion of a vertebra—from a centrum into a pedicle and possibly into a lamina. The supporting structure is rapidly depleted, and pathologic fractures even to the degree of out and out compression with abrupt kyphosis or scoliosis may occur. These changes, of course, produce symptoms and signs which might readily be misinterpreted as tuberculous spondylitis.

Dyscrasias of the hemopoietic system such as primary anemias and leukemias or plasma cell myeloma may be manifested in the vertebrae. In any one vertebra the changes found in leukemia or primary anemias may closely simulate those of hemangioma. However, with hemangiomas the changes are confined to one or a few vertebrae, while with the blood dyscrasias they involve a series.

The primary form of plasma cell myeloma has been described as closely simulating the appearance of giant cell tumor (when located in a centrum). The patient's age (over 40 for plasma cell myeloma; usually under that for giant cell tumor) and the difference in response to roentgenotherapy (rapid and immediate in the case of plasma cell myeloma; gradual in the case of giant cell tumor) may serve to differentiate.

Secondary or metastatic lesions of plasma cell myeloma early present the appearance of extensive deossification as seen in hyper-

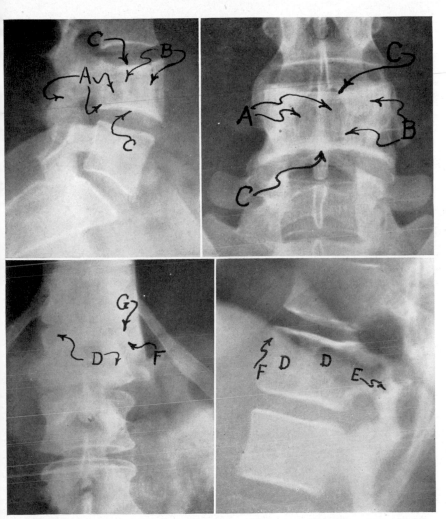

Backache and pain may be attributable to lesions of bones. Hemangiomas **(Figs. 640 and 641, above)** may cause minimal distress, though their presence is usually an accidental observation. They are featured by scattered areas of increased ray transparency, A; coarsened intervening trabeculation scaffolding, B; possibly, evidence of prolonged deficiency of tensile strength—concavity of contour—C (due to pressure of nucleus pulposus). More extensive dissolution of bone, D **(Figs. 642 and 643, below)** prompts consideration of giant cell tumor. Note extension into pedicles, E. Pathologic fractures, F, may occur even to the extent of complete collapse, G, which may be the first sign.

parathyroidism. Later, the individual lesions are more conspicuous, appearing as multiple punched-out lesions with no evidence of bone reaction around them and no evidence of periosteal changes.

Vertebrae are highly susceptible to metastatic involvement. The metastases may be secondary to any one of a variety of primary lesions. In females, most frequently the primary neoplasm is located in the breast. The metastatic lesions may be osteolytic and therefore difficult to discern or may be osteoblastic (particularly following menopause). In males, the most frequent location of the primary neoplasm is the prostate. These metastatic lesions are usually osteoblastic.

A variety of locations of the primary neoplasm must be considered when metastases are suspected: malignancies of the kidney or adrenal, testicles, thyroid or lungs and even of the gastro-intestinal tract. Lymphoblastomas may produce similar defects.

All metastatic lesions are featured by their multiplicity; by involvement of many parts of many bones. They involve cancellous structure in particular. They may produce so much destruction as to cause collapse of one or more centra, with resultant kyphosis or scoliosis of abrupt angulation. They may produce much pain and possibly embarrassment to the cord or nerve roots.

Thus these lesions of the bones must be included in an analysis of the cause of painful movements of the spine.

Chordomas

SYNONYMS: Chordoblastoma, chordocarcinoma, chordo-epithelioma, ecchondrosis or ecchordosis physaliphora, malignancy of fetal notochord.

ROENTGEN CRITERIA

EARLY STAGES

Soft tissues: Ray-transparent tumefaction in midline position.

Apophyseal joints: Uninvolved.

Amphi-arthrodial joints: Centra—possibly, slight erosions of anterior or posterior surfaces. Articular disks—possibly, slightly widened.

Sacro-iliac joints: Possibly, slightly expanded.

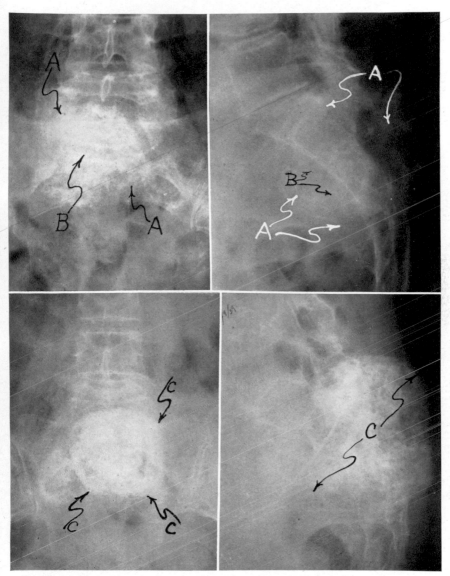

Figs. 644–647.—As in peripheral joints, malignant bone tumors—osteochondrosarcomas—may cause symptoms in spinal joints. Speckling of calcification, A, in continuity with bone outline points to this type of lesion. Preponderance of ray transparency (i.e., cartilage), B, in the tumor points to malignancy (vs. osteochondroma). **Figs. 646 and 647 (below).**—Findings after extensive roentgen therapy. Note calcifications, C.

Regional skeleton: Possibly, erosions of sella turcica, clivus, sphenoid sinus, etc.

LATER STAGES

Soft tissues: Ray-transparent tumefaction (occasionally containing calcific speckling), possibly of considerable dimensions with resultant deviation in position of structures such as intestines, ureters, kidneys, etc., when in the lower spine, or of the posterior wall of the pharynx or esophagus when in the upper spine.

Regional joints: Expansion—erosions; possibly, conspicuous destruction of bones.

CORROBORATIVE ROENTGEN CRITERIA: Chest studies may indicate metastases. Studies of skeleton may indicate distant metastases; in those of upper spine, encephalography may indicate deviation of third ventricle.

INCIDENCE

Age: Seldom disturbing prior to fourth decade (one case in day-old infant).

Sex: Reported in males approximately twice as often as in females.

Location: Sacral region involved in about two thirds; in other third, usually region of sphenoid (i.e., dorsum sellae).

Trauma: Related in about one third of cases involving lower spine.

HISTORY: Symptoms variable, depending on location of tumor; they develop slowly.

When in sacral region, possibly background of trauma; otherwise, local pain or distress for months, usually followed by radiating pains into buttocks or over sciatic distribution. Later, paralytic and trophic changes, lower extremities; possibly, interference with defecation or urination and with sitting position.

When in the region of the sphenoid, first evidence may be of headache and possibly dizziness, nausea and vomiting. Later, progressive failure of vision and diplopia; possibly, cranial nerve palsies; possibly. pressure phenomena in nasopharynx—dysphagia.

When located elsewhere, likely aching and segmental neuritis. Later, signs of cord compression; possibly, pressure on adjacent organs.

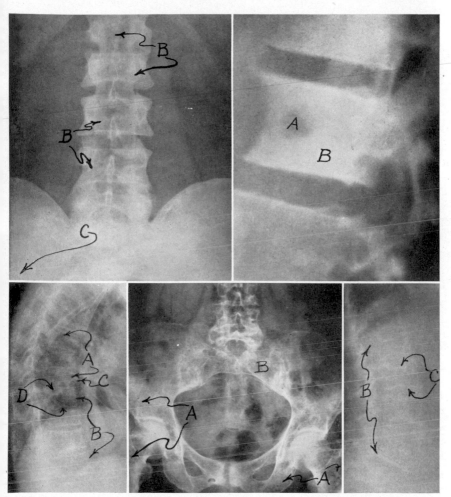

Figs. 648 and 649 (above).—Various types of backache may be produced by metastatic lesions. They may be osteolytic, A, or osteoblastic, B. One or a few vertebrae may be involved or practically the entire series, together with infiltrative osteolytic or osteoblastic mottling in sacrum and ilium, C. **Figs. 650–652 (below).**—Backache may be produced by osteolytic lesions of plasma cell myeloma, usually found in older persons. Numerous punched-out lesions, A; generalized deossification, B (as found in older persons with reduced activity); possibly, compression, C; biconcavities, D (comparable to those found in hyperparathyroidism).

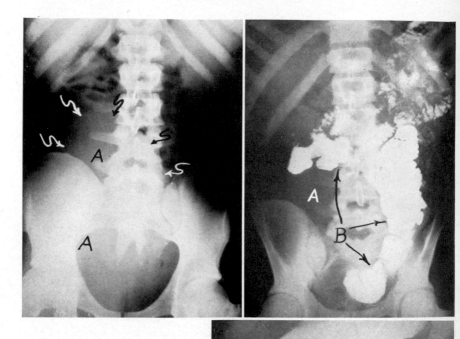

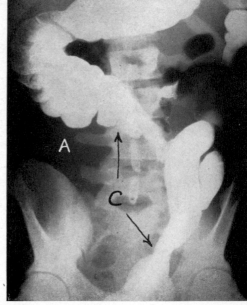

Figs. 653–655, and Figs. 656–659 (facing page).—Chordoma, sacral region. Note ray-transparent mass, A. These tumors are usually detected by indirect evidence: deviations of small intestine, B; colon, C; and ureters, D. They may produce erosion of centra, sacrum or ilium, E. Though slow-growing, they have definite malignant characteristics, as established by ultimate metastases (see Figs. 658 and 659).

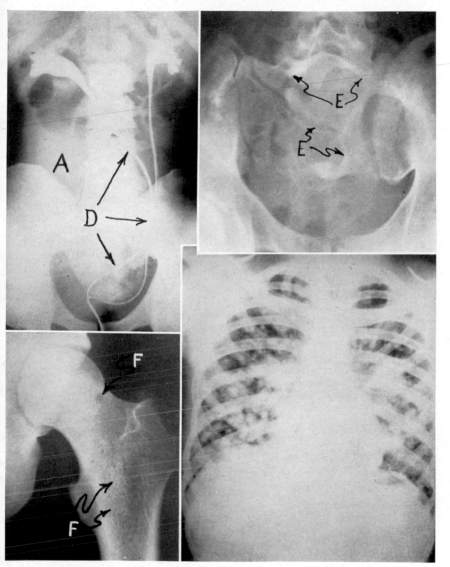

Figs. 656 and 657 (above).—See legend, facing page. **Fig. 658 (left below).**—Chordoma metastases to skeleton, F. **Fig. 659 (right below).**—Chordoma metastases to lungs.

PHYSICAL FINDINGS: When in sacral region, likely palpable mass (on rectal examination); possibly, evidence of blood or mucus in rectum; possibly, trophic changes or actual paralysis, lower extremities.

When in sphenoid, possibly papilledema, optic atrophy; possibly, evidence of cranial nerve paralysis; possibly, bulging of one or both eyes, proptosis, etc., possibly, hemiplegia or paraplegia and signs of increased intracranial pressure.

When located elsewhere, possibly signs of spinal cord compression with block; possibly, palpable tumor.

LABORATORY FINDINGS: Usually uninformative.

CLINICAL COURSE: Slowly progressive in growth; great tendency to recur following removal; metastasis late; average duration of life, two years or less after appearance of symptoms, with no treatment.

BIBLIOGRAPHY

ADSON, A. W.; KERNOHAN, J. W., AND WOLTMAN, H. W.: Cranial and Cervical Chordomas, Arch. Neurol. & Psychiat. 33:247–261, 1935.

ALPERS, B. J., AND PANCOAST, H. K.: Haemangioma of Vertebrae, Surg., Gynec. & Obst. 55:374–376, 1932.

ANDREWS, J. R.: Spheno-Occipital Chordoma of Unusual Radiosensitivity, Radiology 39:478–479, 1942.

BAILEY, P., AND BAGDASAR, D.: Intracranial Chordoblastoma, Am. J. Path. 5:439–450, 1929.

———, AND BUCY, P. C.: Cavernous Hemangioma of Vertebrae, J. A. M. A. 92:1748–1751, 1929.

CAMP, J. D.; ADSON, A. W., AND SHUGRUE, J. J.: Roentgenographic Findings Associated with Tumors of Spinal Column, Spinal Cord and Associated Tissues, Am. J. Cancer 17:348–372, 1933.

———, AND GOOD, C. A., Jr.: Roentgenologic Diagnosis of Tumors Involving the Sacrum, Radiology 31:398–403, 1938.

CARMICHAEL, F. A., Jr.; HELWIG, F. C., AND WHEELER, J. H.: Cranial Chordoma, Am. J. Surg. 55:583–587, 1942.

COTTON, A.: Giant Cell Tumor of Spine, Am. J. Roentgenol. 20:18–24, 1928.

FLETCHER, E. M.; WOLTMAN, H. W., AND ADSON, A. W.: Sacrococcygeal Chordomas, Arch. Neurol. & Psychiat. 33:283–299, 1935.

GARDNER, W. J., AND TURNER, O.: Cranial Chordomas; Clinical & Pathologic Study, Arch. Surg. 42:411–425, 1941.

GREENWOOD, J., Jr.: Space-Occupying Lesions of Spinal Canal, Texas State J. Med. 36:305–310, 1940.

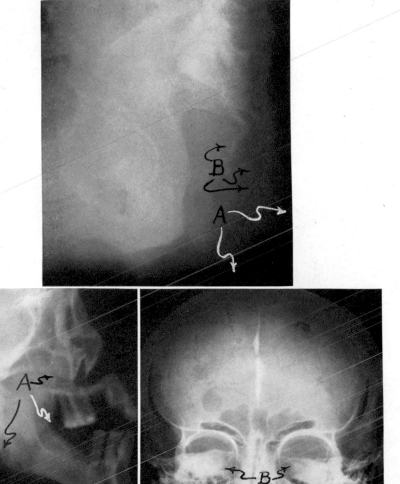

Aberrant notochord tissues and malignancies arising therefrom are most frequently located either at the sacral extremity **(Fig. 660, above)** or at the cephalic extremity, regional to the sella turcica **(Figs. 661 and 662, below)**. Note ray transparency of mass, A, and erosion of contiguous bone, B.

GRIEVE, W. E.: Giant Cell Tumor of Vertebrae, Northwest Med. 33:81–84, 1934.

HASS, G. M.: Chordomas of Cranium and Cervical Portion of Spine; Review of Literature with Report of Case, Arch. Neurol. & Psychiat. 32:300–327, 1934.

JENKINSON, E. L.; HUNTER, A. F., AND ROBERTS, E. W.: Giant Cell Tumor of Vertebrae; 2 Cases, Am. J. Roentgenol. 40:344–347, 1938.

KELLY, L. C.: Vertebral Hemangioma with Neurologic Symptoms, New York State J. Med. 40:1607–1612, 1940.

LEWIS, D.: Primary Giant Cell Tumors of Vertebrae, J. A. M. A. 83:1224–1229, 1924.

MAREK, F. M.: Aneurysm of Abdominal Aorta with Manifestations Simulating Pott's Disease, Bull. Hosp. Joint Dis. 1:51–56, 1940.

MURPHY, G. W.: Giant Cell Tumor of Spine, Am. J. Roentgenol. 34:386–394, 1935.

PEERS, J. H.: Spino-Occipital Chordoma, Am. J. Cancer 32:221–226, 1938.

RICHARDS, V., AND KING, D.: Chordoma, Surgery 8:409–423, 1940.

SANTOS, J. V.: Giant Cell Tumor of Spine, Ann. Surg. 91:37–43, 1930.

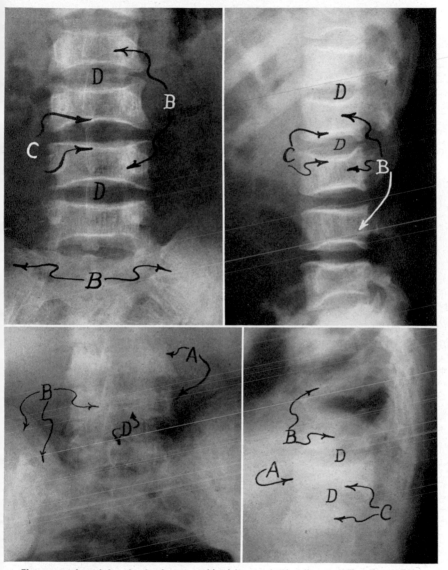

Figs. 663 and 664 (above).—Lumbar spine in blood dyscrasia (sickle cell anemia). **Figs. 665 and 666 (below).**—Lumbar spine in osteitis deformans. Note evidence of diminished tensile strength: flattening with increased horizontal diameters, *A;* coarsened trabeculation pattern, *B;* slight eburnation, *C;* biconcavity (i.e., expansion of disks), *D.*

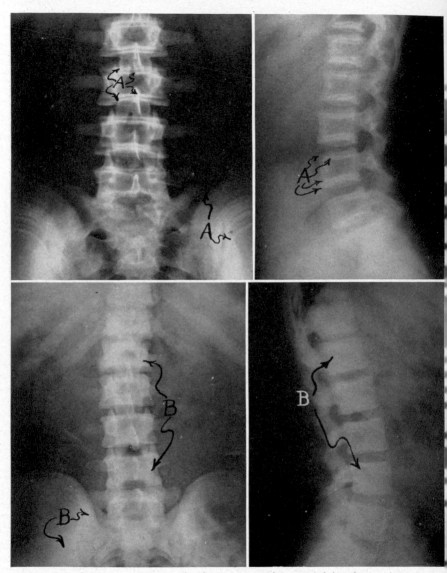

Coarsened trabeculations such as those found with osseous replacement and deossification phenomena must not be confused with interval deposits of heavy metals such as lead and phosphorus (A in **Figs. 667 and 668, above)** or with widespread osteosclerosis such as that found in chronic fluoride poisoning (B in **Figs. 669 and 670, below).**

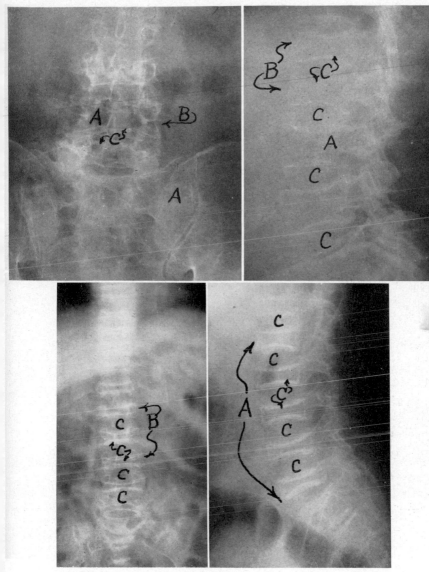

Diminished tensile strength may be caused by hyperparathyroidism **(Figs. 671 and 672, above).** Note marked ray transparency of bones, A; compression, B; biconcavity, C. General appearance may resemble senescent osteo-arthropathy, though eburnations, spurs and the older age of patients with the latter should aid in distinguishing. Similar changes may be found with deficiencies of bone formation such as osteogenesis imperfecta **(Figs. 673 and 674, below).**

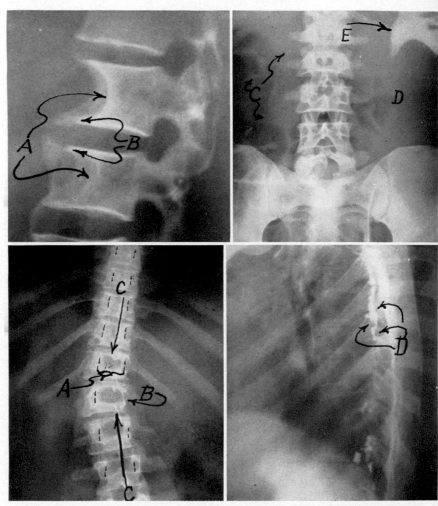

Backache and spinal joint pain may be caused by tumefactions in the region of the spine. **Fig. 675 (left above).**—Aneurysm. Note pulsation erosion, involving midosseous portions, A, but sparing extremities, B, which are cushioned by articular cartilage. **Fig. 676 (right above).**—Paraspinal (perinephritic) abscess. Outline of kidney and iliopsoas muscle on normal side, C, and their obliteration on side of the inflammatory lesion, D; deviation of kidney, E. Similar deviation may be caused by soft tissue neoplasm which may cause backache. Such a lesion may be distinguished from abscess by outline of soft tissue tumefaction *without* obliteration of muscle and kidney outlines (i.e., signs of inflammation). **Figs. 677 and 678 (below).**—Intraspinal tumors may cause backache. Pressure may be indicated by abrupt variation in interpedicular spacing, A; complete erosion of a pedicle, B, and scoliosis, C, or more definitely by filling defects in bolus of radiopaque medium, D (case of multiple neurofibromas).

General Bibliography

ALLISON, N., AND GHORMLEY, R. K.: Diagnosis of Joint Disease (New York: William Wood & Company, 1931).

BENNETT, G. A.; WAINE, H., AND BAUER, W.: Changes in the Knee Joint at Various Ages (New York: Commonwealth Fund, 1942).

BRAILSFORD, J. F.: Radiology of Bones and Joints (New York: William Wood & Company, 1934).

CODMAN, E. A.: The Shoulder (Boston: Thomas Todd Company, 1934).

COMROE, B. I.: Arthritis and Allied Conditions (Philadelphia: Lea & Febiger, 1940).

ELY, L.: Chronic Arthritis, M. Rec. 101:223–227, 1922.

FERGUSON, A. B.: Roentgen Diagnosis of Extremities and Spine, in Annals of Roentgenology (New York: Paul B. Hoeber, Inc., 1941), Vol. XVII.

FISHER, A. G. T.: Chronic (Non-Tuberculous) Arthritis (New York: The Macmillan Company, 1929).

FORESTIER, J., AND ROBERT, P.: X-Ray Diagnosis in Chronic Arthritis, Proc. Roy. Soc. Med. 33:707–724, 1940.

GESCHICKTER, C. F., AND COPELAND, M. M.: Tumors of Bone, Internat. S. Dig. 10:323–343, 1930.

GHORMLEY, R. K.: Pathologic Changes in Disease of Joints, Am. J. Roentgenol. 29:729–735, 1933.

GOLDEN, R.: Diagnostic Roentgenology (New York: Thos. Nelson & Sons, 1941).

GOLDHAMER, K.: X-Ray Therapy of Chronic Arthritis (Including X-Ray Diagnosis of the Disease), (Quincy, Ill.: Radiologic Review Publishing Co., 1941).

HENCH, P. S.: Acute and Chronic Arthritis, in Nelson's Loose Leaf Surgery (New York: Thomas Nelson & Sons, 1935), Vol. III, pp. 104–175 H.

HOLMES, G. W.: Roentgen Interpretation (6th ed.; Philadelphia: Lea & Febiger, 1941).

JORDAN, E. P.: Differential Diagnosis of Arthritis from Standpoint of Pathology, J. Lab. & Clin. Med. 22:6–11, 1936.

KNAGGS, R. L.: Inflammatory and Toxic Diseases of Bone (New York: William Wood & Company, 1926).

KÖHLER, A.: Roentgenology: The Borderlands of the Normal and Early Pathological in Skiagram (2d ed.; London: Baillière, Tindall & Cox, 1935).

MARGOLIS, H. M.: Conquering Arthritis (New York: The Macmillan Company, 1931).

MONROE, R. T.: Chronic Arthritis, in Oxford Loose-Leaf Medicine (New York: Oxford University Press, 1939), ch. xv, pp. 367–404.

NICHOLS, E. H., AND RICHARDSON, F. L.: Arthritis Deformans, J. M. Research 21:149, 1909.

PANCOAST, H. K.; PENDERGRASS, E. P., AND SCHAEFFER, J. P.: The Head and Neck in Roentgen Diagnosis (Springfield, Ill.: Charles C Thomas, Publisher, 1940).

PEMBERTON, R.: Arthritis and Rheumatoid Conditions (2d ed.; Philadelphia: Lea & Febiger, 1935).

RIGLER, L. G.: Outline of Roentgen Diagnosis (Philadelphia: J. B. Lippincott Company, 1938).

SANTE, L. R.: Manual of Roentgenological Technique (9th ed.; Ann Arbor, Mich.: Edwards Bros., 1942).

SCOTT, S. G.: Adolescent Spondylitis or Ankylosing Spondylitis (New York: Oxford University Press, 1942).

TAYLOR, G. D.; FERGUSON, A. B.; KASABACH, H., AND DAWSON, M. H.: Roentgenologic Observations on Various Types of Chronic Arthritis, Arch. Int. Med. 57:979–998, 1936.

Index

NOTE.—Asterisk (*) indicates reference to page of illustrations.

K

Kidneys: abscess, confusing spinal picture, 308*; disease, periarticular swelling with, 219*
Kienböck's disease: 84, 87*; in wrist, after trauma, 99*
Kilovoltage: high, evaluation, 18, 19, 21*; for joints of extremities, 20; sensitization curve and, 20
Kissing erosions: 161, 167*
Klippel-Feil syndrome: 243*
Knee: anatomy, 29*; Baker's cyst in, 219*; calcific deposits after trauma, 214*; in gonococcic arthritis, 177*; in hemophilia, 127*; hemorrhagic arthropathy in, 125 f.*; infectious arthritis via cellulitis in, 187*; kilovoltage for, 19*; with melorheostosis leri, 203*; milkman's, 102; in mixed arthropathy, 160*; neoplasms in, 201*; normal, diodrast in, 219*; osteo-arthropathy after removal of semilunar cartilage, 114*; osteochondritic sequestration in, 95*; pneumoarthrography, 107*; in rheumatoid arthritis, 148 f.*, 153*, 155*; senescent arthropathy in, 122*; sesamoids in, 49*; in staphylococcic arthritis, 185*; synovioma of, 207, 208*; with transverse myelitis, 137*, 138*; traumatic hemorrhagic osteo-arthropathy in, 128, 129*; in tuberculous arthritis in youth, 166*
Köhler's disease: 84, 87, 89
König's disease: 93 ff.
Kyphosis: adolescentium, 244 ff.; with bone-cartilage pathology, 245*; dorsalis juvenilis, 244 ff.; from lesions of anterior horns or efferent nerves, 271*; from mesenchymal defects, 231*

L

Lead: in spine, 306*; in sites of bone growth, 220*
Legg's disease: 74 ff.
Leprosy: ainhum resembling, 215*; arthropathy of, 134 ff., 139*; fingers in, 139*; rheumatoid lesions comparable to, 158*; toes in, 139*
Leriche's atrophy: 102 ff., 108*
Ligaments, calcification in: in Pellegrini-Stieda's disease, 214*; posttraumatic, 110*
Limbus: vs. osteochondropathy, 249*

Lipomas: 201*; in peripheral joints, 199
Liver: in juvenile rheumatoid arthritis, 147*
Lordosis, lumbar: in early rheumatoid arthritis, 275*; with spondylolisthesis, 240*
Lumbarization: 242*
Lungs: with allergic arthritis, 143*; chordoma metastases to, 303*; with sarcoid, 216*

M

Macrodactyly: 48*
Madelung's deformity: 43*; from trauma, 90*
Marie-Bamberger's disease: 217*
Marie-Strümpell's disease: 274 ff.; confused with osteo-arthropathy, 263*
Melorheostosis Leri: 203*
Meniscus: calcifications, 221*; cyst in, 204*; deranged lateral, 107*
Mesothelioma: 205 ff.
Metacarpal: in congenital syphilis, 58*; stunted from epiphyseal failure, 48*; synarthrosis of, 41*
Metaphyses: in active rickets, 63*; in juvenile osteochondropathy of hip, 75*; in scurvy, 71*
Metastases: from chordoma, 303*; to lungs, 208*; suggesting "rheumatism," 210*; to vertebrae, 296
Metatarsal: atavistic, 114*; bone-cartilage damage, 85*; in leprosy, 139*; osteochondropathy of, 84 ff.
Morbus coxae senilis: 117 ff.
Muscle atrophy: in inflammatory rheumatoid arthritis, 155*; from poliomyelitis, 215*
Muscle bundles: with neoplasms, 203*; in tuberculous arthritis of hip, 163*
Myelitis, transverse: hip with, 138*; knee in, 137 f.*
Myelocele: 225*
Myelography: of prolapsed disk, 258*, 259*
Myeloma, plasma cell: confused with abnormal centra, 227*; confused with spinal osteo-arthropathy, 269*; spine in, 294, 299*
Myositis ossificans: 203*

N

Navicular: bipartite, 105*; —contrasted to fracture, 47*; fracture, 105*; osteo-chondropathy of, 89*